Welcome

Well, well, well! Guess what? You've officially stepped into the thrilling,
enchanting realm of pregnancy! Get ready for a rollercoaster ride filled
with belly bumps, cravings, and the occasional existential crisis.
Oh, and don't forget the radiant glow and superhuman sense of smell - it's
like having a spidey sense for takeout! Now, buckle up because this book
is your ticket to surviving the wild ride ahead.

Question 1: Are you prepared to embrace the epic transformation that's
about to turn your body and life into a surreal carnival of surprises? Get
ready to trade your regular pants for a collection of stretchy wonders!

Question 2: Ever find yourself pondering the mysteries of pregnancy, like
how can something the size of a peanut create a craving for pickles
dunked in chocolate? And oh, navigating mood swings that rival a
daytime soap opera? Fear not, we've got the cheat codes!

Question 3: Curious about the baby-building extravaganza happening
inside your belly? From barely a poppy seed to a whole watermelon (not
literally), we've got the scoop on how your mini-human is cooking in
there.

Question 4: Are you secretly Googling "Can I eat this while pregnant?"
every time you sit down for a meal? Or wondering if the discomfort
you're experiencing is just part of the magical experience? Buckle up,
we've got tips to keep you and your little sidekick healthy and
comfortable.

And guess what? If your response to any of these questions was a
resounding "heck yes!" then say hello to your newfound BFF.
Within these pages, you'll not only uncover the secrets of pregnancy but
also indulge in tales of superhero-like cravings, tender moments, and
wizard-level advice that'll make you feel like a pregnancy pro.
So, let's flip the pages and dive headfirst into this wacky and wonderful
adventure together!

Ready, set, baby bump!

The first 3 weeks of your pregnancy

When you are, but you are not, but you are pregnant... Let me explain.

All right, hold on to your belly bump because here's the crazy truth about those first two weeks of a typical 40-week pregnancy—it's like you're on a pre-pregnancy vacation!

Seriously, you're not officially "preggo" yet. It's like a sneak peek before the real show begins. Picture this: You're planning a 40-week baby extravaganza, but the bun is still in the oven, and the oven is still preheating! It's like your uterus is setting the stage for the most epic production of your life.

Now, the hilarious part is that around the 14th day of your typical 28-day cycle, there's this thing called "Ovulation Day!" It's like your egg is putting on its best party dress, waiting to meet its dance partner—
a super eager sperm!
But hold your horses, Mr. Sperm! You're a little early to the baby-making ball. You still have to wait for that egg-cellent moment. It's like the sperm is practicing its dance moves while the egg is like, "Not yet, buddy, not yet!"

Week two is all about the follicular phase, which is like the pre-game before the ovulation party! And hey, if you have a 28-day cycle, your egg-scapade happens around the 14th day of your cycle. That's when the real baby-making dance begins.

So, imagine you're finally in week three, and guess what?
You're officially pregnant! Ta-da!
Easy-peasy-lemon-sqeezy!

To sum it up, those first two weeks of "pregnancy" are like the sneakiest countdown ever. It's like the warm-up act before the main event. You're prepping the nursery, but the star of the show is still rehearsing backstage.
So, buckle up, because once the real pregnancy party starts, it's going to be a wild ride!

How you might feel in the first 2-weeks?

During those early weeks of pregnancy (and heck, maybe even up to the third if your cycle is playing hard to get), your body is like, "Nah, no signs of pregnancy yet, folks!" It's because the magical moment of conception, where the bun gets into the oven, hasn't happened just yet.

Your body is transforming, preparing for the creation of a tiny human, and major changes are happening inside it:
· Around two weeks after the first day of your last period, something truly magical happens in your body! One of your ovaries lovingly releases a tiny egg cell.
· This little wonder embarks on a journey down one of your fallopian tubes, eagerly awaiting a chance to meet a sperm prince and create new life.

 It's an extraordinary process that brings the potential for a beautiful new beginning.

So, don't fret if you're not feeling any baby kicks or cravings for pickles and ice cream – it's all on its way!
Hang in there, and soon enough, you'll start experiencing the wild roller coaster of pregnancy symptoms in the second half of your first month. Your baby's little adventure is just getting started!

What are the early telltale signs, that you are expecting a bundle of joy?

Oh, the first few weeks of pregnancy can be like a sneaky little mystery! You might not even have a clue that something magical is happening inside you because it's just too early to notice any telltale signs.
No worries, though – it's totally natural. Heck, by the third week, you might not even have conceived yet!

But fear not, the universe has its ways of dropping hints.
One of the early signs you might notice is the absence of your regular period. That's like the universe's way of giving you a little nudge. And around that same time or a bit later, you might start noticing other curious signals of pregnancy.
Some folks might experience what's called implantation bleeding – a light spotting that happens when a "cluster of cells" (not a zygote anymore, but a blastocyst!) snuggles up in the cozy lining of your uterus.

Now, here's the funny twist – this implantation bleeding doesn't happen to all pregnant women, so it's like a secret handshake for some.
And, guess what? It can easily be mistaken for your regular period, playing a little trick on you.
So, if you're keeping an eye out for the signs, remember to look for the absence of your period and keep an ear out for any other early pregnancy clues.
The magic might be brewing, and you'll soon be on an incredible journey of discovery!

Possible symptoms of pregnancy
(where unicorns and rainbows are nowhere to be seen)

Oh, the first month of pregnancy is like a fun-filled roller coaster of surprises! As your little bun starts to grow, it might send some playful signals your way. Here are some of the quirky signs you could encounter:

Bloating: Yep, you might feel like you swallowed a helium balloon! Enjoy the whimsical ride, my lighter-than-air friend!

Gas: Oh yes, even a mom-to-be can have some toots! Blame it on those hormonal acrobatics and the little life starting to bloom inside you.

Fatigue: Get ready for some extra Zzz's, because growing a tiny human is no easy task! Feeling like you could nap anytime, anywhere is just your body's way of saying, "Take it easy, superhero!"

Breast tenderness: Ouch! Your lovely ladies might feel a bit tender and sensitive like they're getting ready for a grand performance as the best milk bar in town.

Fluctuating mood: Ah, the emotional roller coaster! One minute you're laughing, the next you're crying over cute puppy videos. Blame it on those hormones having a dance party.

Frequent urination: You might find yourself running to the bathroom more often than usual. Your little passenger is taking up space, after all!

Remember, every pregnancy is unique, so not all these signs will be a part of your journey. But if you notice some of these quirks, it could be your body's way of saying, "Congratulations, you're on the baby-making adventure!".

Embrace the journey, and enjoy every moment (even if you cannot trust your own farts...).

Where are you on the pregnancy journey?

Knowing where you stand in your pregnancy journey is super crucial, both for you and your doctor. They'll use this intel to keep a close eye on your baby's growth and development and also to make sure you're in the pink of health by scheduling those prenatal tests.

So, let's break it down – pregnancy is divided into three awesomely named trimesters:

Weeks 1 to 12 - *"The Barf-O-Rama Adventure: Nausea and Morning Sickness Take the Stage!"*
It's like the opening act of an amazing show, where everything starts to take shape, and the adventure is just getting started.

Weeks 13 to 27 - *"Cravings Galore: The Hunt for the Strangest Food Combinations Begins!"*
By now, your little one is growing, and it's like a fantastic middle part of the journey – full of kicks, flutters, and some amazing baby milestones.

Weeks 28 to 40 (and beyond) - *"Waddle Fest 3000: The Art of Elegant Movement While Carrying a Watermelon-Sized Belly!"*
This is the grand finale, the last stretch (yep, stretchmark as well) where you're eagerly counting down to meet your baby. Things might get a bit cramped in there, but it's all part of the magical experience.

Calculating your due date is like a fascinating baby math puzzle!

So, doctors have this funky rule, and they start counting the pregnancy weeks from the first day of your last period.
It's like they're playing "Guess the Due Date" with Mother Nature.

Here's how it's done:

Starting Point:
The first step is to figure out the first day of your last menstrual period (LMP). It's like the initial piece of the puzzle.

Counting Days:
From the first day of your LMP, doctors will add 280 days (or 40 weeks) to get an estimated due date. Keep in mind that this is just an estimate, and babies have their own sense of timing!

Ultrasound Confirmation:
As your pregnancy progresses, your doctor might use ultrasound scans to measure the baby's growth and development. These scans can provide a more accurate due date or confirm the one calculated based on your LMP.

Adjustments for Irregular Cycles:
If you have irregular menstrual cycles or are unsure about the date of your LMP, your doctor might use other methods like measuring the size of the uterus or analyzing hormone levels to estimate the due date.

Remember, Babies Have Their Own Plans:
It's essential to understand that the due date is an estimate, not an exact science. Babies can arrive a bit earlier or later than expected, and that's perfectly normal. Only about 5% of babies are born on their due date!

Week 4

Congratulations, you've got a teeny-tiny poppy seed guest chilling in your womb!

They may be just 2mm long, but trust me, they've already mastered the art of rapid growth. Picture them hanging out in their exclusive amniotic sac, enjoying their cushy, fluid-filled castle – the fanciest hot tub in town!

And let's not forget their personal chef, the yolk sac, whipping up all the gourmet meals they need. Bon appétit, little seedling!

Well, while you're busy adjusting to the wondrous world of pregnancy, your little tenant inside is pulling off a full-scale construction project! It's like they've got their own tiny crew, building away inside your womb. First, they set up camp in the luxurious uterine wall after a long journey, making it their official embryo headquarters.

And boy, are they ambitious!

They're dividing cells left and right, forming layers like they're building a skyscraper. They've got big plans for this little body they're creating – a fully functional nervous system, a sturdy skeleton, jacked-up muscles, and all the fancy organs you can think of. They're even hiring an interior designer to work on the skin – fashionista from the get-go!

But that's not all!

The baby-to-be is also making some real-estate deals, forming the placenta to connect with you, the gracious host. It's like a bridge between your worlds, and they're making sure it's in a prime location – right on the uterus wall!

Oh, and don't forget the umbilical cord, the baby's personal line to room service! They're making sure it's top-notch, slowly growing over time. Now, for some extra coziness, they've got a little DIY project going on inside the yolk sac, creating amniotic fluid to serve as a cushy, protective buffer for their stay.

And guess what? The brain and spine aren't left out either! They're crafting the neural tube, the ultimate building block for a genius-level brain and a spine to keep everything in check.

It's like a tiny construction wonderland in there, and they're just getting started!

Your body

Ah, the mystical signs of pregnancy reveal themselves during the fourth week! Some moms-to-be get to experience mild cramping and spotting – like a secret code signaling the arrival of the fertilized egg to its cozy nest in the uterus.

And guess what?
Your body has got the hormone factory up and running! The superstar hormone, hCG, is now making its grand entrance. It's like the conductor of a magical orchestra, instructing your ovaries to take a well-deserved vacation from releasing eggs, effectively stopping your monthly period – ta-da!

But that's not all; it's also pulling the strings on other hormone production like estrogen and progesterone.

How you might feel in the 4th week?

Ah, the glamorous life of a mom-to-be!

Welcome to the fourth week of pregnancy, where you get to experience a series of delightful surprises!

Embrace Your New Superpower: Fatigue Unleashed!
Surprise! It's not just for mornings! It can strike anytime, like a mischievous ninja. Some lucky ladies get a mild version, while others get the full-blown vomiting extravaganza – like an Olympic sport of nausea! But don't fret, you're not alone in this queasy adventure; around 80 percent of pregnant women get to join the "nausea club." The silver lining? As the second trimester knocks on the door, this unwelcome guest often decides to peace out!

Pregnancy Fountain Flow: A Clear, Sticky Tale from Down Below
Next up, we've got the light-colored vaginal discharge. It's totally normal, with a sticky consistency, and should be clear or light in color. No worries, your body is just prepping the welcome mat for the little one. However, if any weird odors, itching, or pain crash the party, make sure to inform your pregnancy bouncer, AKA your doctor.

The Progesterone Plunge: Special Delivery - Extreme Exhaustion

You'll feel like you've run a marathon after just a few steps – your body is working overtime to create a magical world for the baby.

Thanks, progesterone hormone, for this extra-special gift of exhaustion! But wait, there's more! Feeling like a sleepy sloth could also be a sign of low iron levels, leading to the epic battle of anemia. Talk to your doctor about the secret potion of iron supplementation to keep you energized throughout this wild journey.

Belly Bloated Extravaganza: Your Body's Pre-Baby Party

It's like a sneak preview of the nine-month-old baby party your body is hosting. Get ready to feel a little puffy, especially in the lower abdomen – your uterus is expanding its real estate like a pro!

Emotional Pendulum Championship: Hormones in the Spotlight!

Get ready to experience the wildest swings of emotions, like a championship pendulum competition! Hormones are having a grand old time, cranking up the intensity of your feelings, and they have a special love for the first and third trimesters – go figure!

Milkshake Magic: Gourmet Kitchen Prep for Newborn Feasts

Welcome to the magical world of breast tenderness in the fourth week! It's like your lovely bosom is gearing up for its superstar role in feeding the little one-to-be. Get ready for some serious action as the milk glands start multiplying like rabbits, and the fat layer is having a blast, turning your breasts into luxurious, plump pillows!

It's the ultimate preparation, like a top-notch gourmet kitchen getting ready to serve up the best milkshakes in town! But be warned, with all this exciting growth happening, your breasts might feel a little sensitive and swollen (ouch!).

Spotlight on "Implementation Spotting": The Sneak Peek Surprise
Don't forget about the "light bleeding or spotting" show! It's like a magic trick called "implementation spotting," where some women get to witness a little spotting action. It's just a small surprise package, as long as it lasts for two days or less. Anything more or any other weird symptoms, and it's time to call your personal pregnancy superhero – your doctor!

So, buckle up for this rollercoaster ride of unexpected sensations, and remember, no two pregnancies are the same. It's like a personalized experience designed just for you!
Enjoy the journey, supermom!

It's time to take care of yourself and your growing little superstar

Healthy eating is the name of the game!
Load up on iron-rich foods like spinach and cereal to keep anemia at bay. Don't forget the protein party – milk, cheese, and yogurt are your go-to pals for building strong bones in that little one.

It's time to kick those bad habits to the curb!
Quit smoking and bid farewell to alcohol – water and other healthy drinks are the new cool kids on the block. They'll help you avoid premature birth and birth defects like a pro!

Avoid secondhand smoke!
It's not just about you anymore; your little one deserves a smoke-free environment. Stay away from secondhand smoke, as it can cause all sorts of complications like low birth weight, miscarriage, and ectopic pregnancy.
Your baby will thank you later!

Embrace the zen!

Take a deep breath and relax – stress is not your friend right now. Keep those stress levels low, like a master of tranquility. Your well-being is crucial for a smooth pregnancy journey.

Stay active (with doctor's approval)

If you've been an active superhero before pregnancy, you may continue exercising with your doctor's approval. Moderate physical activity is recommended throughout your pregnancy journey.
But hey, if you were a couch potato before, no worries!
Talk to your doctor about simple exercises suitable for pregnancy, like swimming, walking, or stretching. Keeping your body in tip-top shape is essential for the incredible effort of pregnancy and childbirth.

Folic acid is like the superstar of your pregnancy show!

It's the superhero B vitamin that's got your baby's neural tube covered – that's right, their future brain and spinal cord! So, here's the deal – by taking folic acid before the baby-making extravaganza and during those early trimester shenanigans, you're giving your little one the ultimate protection against pesky neural tube defects. It's like putting up a force field of awesomeness!

So, there you have it – a guide to rocking week 4 of pregnancy like a pro! Take care of yourself and your little bun in the oven.

You've got this, supermom!

Week 5 – 2nd month– 1st Trymester

Ahoy, future parents! Welcome to the week 5.

At the 5th week of pregnancy, the presence of a gestational follicle in the uterine cavity can already be detected during ultrasound. If at this time the yolk follicle is not yet visible inside it, along with the embryo, it will appear in the following week.

Your baby

Look at your little sesame seed superstar, all 2mm of pure cuteness and the shape of a tiny tadpole. The face is getting ready for the grand reveal, with a teeny-tiny nose and adorable little eyes – like a top-secret makeover happening inside your belly!
Don't worry though, those eyes are playing peek-a-boo and staying closed until the big debut at around 28 weeks – baby has got a surprise in store!

Baby Brain and Backbone Bonanza: The Neural Tube Extravaganza!
Get ready to witness the marvel of the century – the neural tube, your baby's very own brain and spine factory, is in full-on action mode!
Think of it as a cutting-edge baby engineering project, complete with all the bells, whistles, and tiny construction hats.

The star of the show making an entrance – drumroll, please – folic acid!
This little gem deserves a standing ovation, so make sure you're taking those 400 micrograms daily. It's like the secret sauce that ensures your baby's nervous system is all jazzed up and ready for success. No nervous system hiccups on this watch – just pure, unadulterated baby brilliance!

Get ready for it to transform into the heart of the party!
Yep, the heart is about to start pumping away like a champ, gearing up for an ultrasound performance that rivals even the best dance moves. Picture it: your baby's heart boogying and grooving during an ultrasound as early as the sixth week. It's like a dance performance that'll have you saying, "Move over, Dancing with the Stars!"

Get ready to have your heart melted by the tiniest, most adorable rhythm in town!

Your baby

Oh wow, your uterus is like a fancy Airbnb for your baby! Only five weeks in, and it's already getting some major renovations.
The placenta and umbilical cord crew are on overtime, delivering all the necessary nutrients to your little tenant. Calcium, folic acid, and other vitamins are like the VIP guests making sure everything goes smoothly in this upscale baby development project.

Keep up the good work, Mama Architect!

How you might feel in the 5th week?

Get ready for this wild ride of emotions and symptoms:

The Unwelcome Wake-Up Call from the Nausea Ninja!
Ah yes, the delightful morning sickness. Still here to make our day...

·When Your Body Decides to Play "Spot the Surprise"
Don't be alarmed if you spot a few drops of blood. But, just to be safe, make sure to let your doctor know about any spotting to avoid any cliffhangers or complications. If things get more serious, rush to your doc immediately!

From Cloud Nine to Waterworks Central – Your Emotional Rollercoaster Pass Has Been Activated!
Buckle up for the emotional rollercoaster! One minute you're on cloud nine, and the next, you might feel like shedding a tear or two. Think of it as a PMS throwback. When your mood is playing tricks on you, try distracting yourself with a walk or blasting your favorite tunes. Embrace the ride and know that it's all part of the pregnancy package.

Pee Party: Welcome to the VIP Restroom Access Club – Pregnancy Edition!
You're now a frequent flyer to the bathroom. The increased blood volume during pregnancy means more fluid to filter, so be prepared for those sudden urges to pee. It might be a bit tiring, but it's all part of the natural process.

When Your Bosom Becomes the Drama Queen of Sensitivity!
Same as in week 4 – we will feel those two friends for a while...

The Progesterone Pillow's VIP Membership – Your Pass to the Land of Naps!
Get ready to be best friends with your bed because you're going to be feeling seriously tired. Blame it on the progesterone party in your body! To catch some quality Z's, avoid caffeine and strenuous activities before bedtime. Stick to a consistent daily schedule, but remember to listen to your body and take breaks when needed. Resting now is like giving yourself and your little one a big high-five for a healthy journey ahead!

When Hormones Think Your Face Is a Canvas for Their Abstract Art!
Oh, joy! Hormonal changes are throwing a party on your skin, and acne is the uninvited guest. Don't worry; it's a common symptom of pregnancy. The good news is, these pesky pimples are likely to make their exit soon after delivery, so hang in there!

When Your Pregnancy Feels Like a Smooth Jazz Playlist Instead of a Heavy Metal Concert!
What if you feel like you're just cruising through this pregnancy ride without any major symptoms? No worries, that's totally normal too! Some women might feel completely normal at this stage, or they might experience symptoms that come and go.

Your abdomen might look pretty much the same or a tad bloated, but no need to fret about extra pounds. If morning nausea and vomiting are your constant companions, you might even lose some weight in the first trimester (we do not recommend pregnancy as a weight loss option – small disclaimer folks).
If you have any questions or concerns about the changes happening (or not happening), don't hesitate to have a chat with your doctor.

Time to be the master chef for your tiny VIP!

Gather your pregnancy pantry heroes for a meal plan that even your little one will applaud!

Uninvited Intruders

Say no to raw or undercooked eggs – those are not invited to the pregnancy feast. And keep the raw or smoked meat at bay – they're not on the guest list either!

Mercury Misfits

Tuna and mackerel may be stylish swimmers, but they're not getting an invite to your pregnancy fiesta.

Cheesy Conundrums

Soft cheeses may be smooth talkers, but their safety record isn't up to par. Unpasteurized dairy products, sushi made with raw fish and oysters, and soft cheeses like brie and feta can cause food-borne illnesses that can put a damper on the pregnancy celebration. Let's keep them off the VIP list.

Bon appétit, superhero mom-to-be!

Hint, hint...!

It's time for some feline wisdom and passing on that litter box duty like a hot potato. No more scooping for you, and here's why: toxoplasmosis, the sneaky little troublemaker.

You see, toxoplasmosis is like that uninvited guest who brings nothing but trouble to the party. It's a parasitic infection that some cats might carry, and it's found in their litter.

But don't worry, we've got a game plan. Delegating this duty to someone else is like putting up a "No Entry" sign for toxoplasmosis. We're on a mission to keep your little one's environment squeaky clean and toxoplasmosis-free.

- First things first, figure out what to consider when choosing the right prenatal care. You want only the best for your little bundle of joy!

- Get ready for your very first pregnancy check-up appointment. Your gynecologist is about to be your new best friend, informing you about future appointments and all those essential tests.

- Speed dial your attending physician and their backup number, not just on your phone but stick it right on the fridge door because you never know when those pregnancy questions will strike.

- When the going gets tough with those annoying cramps and backaches, treat yourself to a warm bath or power nap – Mama deserves some R&R!

- Remember, life can be unpredictable, so find out who to call if your doc decides to go on a tropical vacation right when you need them most.

- Oh, and if you haven't already, it's time to say goodbye to smoking and bid adieu to alcohol. Your baby-to-be deserves a clean and healthy environment from the get-go. Cheers to a smoke-free and alcohol-free life!

Week 6 – 2nd month– 1st Trymester
Your baby

At 6 weeks, your tiny, adorable fetus is like the tiniest intern at a bustling corporation called Life Inc. They're the newbie who just started their gig and they're only about the size of a sprinkle on a cupcake...yum!

Imagine a little poppy seed, lounging around in their comfy uterus office, sipping on some amniotic fluid while trying to figure out the grand plan of becoming a full-fledged human. If we were to throw a party for this microscopic superstar, we'd be serving snacks so small that even an ant would need a magnifying glass to see them.

Get ready to celebrate because this week, our little superstar is hitting a growth spurt that's more exciting than finding extra fries at the bottom of your takeout bag!

Picture this: the neural tube is like a master architect meticulously wrapping up a surprise gift – the future spinal cord – with a ribbon of development. It's like a baby DIY project, only on a cosmic scale!

But wait, there's more, folks!
Our mini Picasso is working on some seriously avant-garde designs – those future peepers and listeners are already crafting their signature looks with small, chic bumps and trendy ear holes. It's like they're plotting to be the most fashionable kid on the block before even making an entrance.

And hold onto your baby booties, because the limbs are getting ready to show off their moves! Those little protuberances on the sides of the embryo?
They're like the embryonic equivalent of jazz hands, getting ready to strut their stuff as the cutest arms and legs in town.

Time to bring out the ultrasound red carpet, because we've got a tiny heartthrob stealing the show! At a heart-pounding tempo of 105 beats per minute, your baby's ticker is like a DJ dropping the hottest beats in the embryonic club scene.

And speaking of scenes, the brain and nervous system are working overtime like a creative genius in a brainstorming session, coming up with all the blueprints for future brilliance.

Now, let's talk lungs – those fabulous, yet-to-be-inflated balloons of life! Between the throat and lungs, these little bronchial buds are busy making plans to become the main bronchi, ready to kickstart the ultimate lung-filling extravaganza – aka your baby's first breath, followed by what will surely be a show-stopping debut cry!

So, there you have it, folks, a week of cosmic construction, runway-worthy developments, and lung-filled anticipation. Your little one is already gearing up to rock this world with style, flair, and a lungful of excitement!

Your body

Ah, welcome to the fabulous sixth week of the baby brewing bonanza! Your body has decided to throw a surprise party and invited all the hormones, changes, and wacky sensations to join the fun.

Smelly Superhero

First off, let's talk about your newfound superpower – the ability to smell things from a mile away. You're like a human bloodhound, detecting scents you never even knew existed. Just remember to steer clear of strong odors unless you want to start a pickle factory in your living room.

Culinary Chaos

Now, speaking of pickles, those cravings might be kicking in like a late-night snack ninja. Suddenly, you're finding yourself craving combinations that even a chef on a reality cooking show would raise an eyebrow at. Ice cream with hot sauce? Why not? Peanut butter and pickles? Sure thing! Embrace the culinary adventure, and who knows, you might discover the next viral food trend!

Snooze Fest

Let's not forget about the unexpected nap attacks. It's like your body has transformed into a cozy hammock, inviting you to take a snooze at the most random moments.

Whether it's during a work meeting or a shopping trip, your body's like, "Hey, let's catch some Z's and dream about baby onesies!"

Emotional Express

Now, onto the magical world of mood swings! One minute you're crying over a heartwarming puppy video, and the next you're laughing uncontrollably at a knock-knock joke. It's like your emotions are on a roller coaster ride with no height requirement.

Bathroom Buddies

Who could forget the bathroom adventures? You and the restroom have become besties, swapping stories and sharing secrets.

But fear not, dear champion of baby-making, because, amidst all these quirks and quips, your body is working its incredible magic to create a tiny human masterpiece.

You're doing an amazing job, and your body deserves a standing ovation – even if you have to do the pee-pee dance to celebrate!

How you might feel in the 6th week?

Yep, get ready for a fantastic round of feeling like a walking dumpster fire.

Here are some delightful contenders:

Sneak Peek or Full Show? Spotting's Mysterious Performance

First up, we've got spotting – the little teaser that keeps you guessing. Just remember, if it's just a sprinkle and not a full-blown paint party, you're likely in the clear. But if your artwork turns into a mural, or if it sticks around like an unwelcome guest, it's time to give your doctor a shout.

Uterus Under Construction: The Contractions Renovation Project

Think of it as the baby version of "Extreme Makeover: Home Edition." Your cozy little baby home is expanding, making room for the precious tenant-to-be. If the cramps are more like a gentle stretching session, you're probably on the right track. But if they start feeling like a full-blown Olympic workout, complete with fever and diarrhea as surprise contestants, it's time to call in the professionals (aka your doctor) for a consultation.

All-Day Drama Queen: Nausea Takes Center Stage

Now, if you've been cruising along nausea-free until now, don't be surprised if this little diva decides to make a dramatic entrance. And let's be clear, it's not just about mornings. Oh no, this star can shine at any hour – morning, noon, or under the moonlit sky.

You're definitely not alone on this roller coaster ride. In fact, as many as 80% of pregnancy performers find themselves grappling with this diva's antics, especially in the opening act of the first trimester. Blame it on hCG, the hormone superstar who's pulling the strings behind the scenes. It's like the conductor of a symphony that occasionally hits a few sour notes.

So, let it be your pregnancy mantra: *"This too shall pass."*

Sure, the nausea might be an unwelcome guest crashing your pregnancy party, but it's temporary.

Handy Tip: Crackers, ginger, salty sticks... all can help a little.

Embrace Your Inner Cat: Power Naps, the New Superpower Against Fatigue

You know those power naps your cat takes? Well, now you're the cat. Quick snoozes during the day are your secret weapon against this fatigue invasion. Plus, who can resist being a professional nap-taker?

Handy Tip: Iron is your knight in shining armor against the villain called Anemia, which loves to disguise itself as chronic exhaustion. So, gobble up those iron-packed foods like a champ – you're not just eating, you're plotting against the fatigue empire.

"Pee-tastic" Odyssey: Bladder Adventures and Kidney Night Shifts

Welcome to the realm of "pee-tastic" adventures – where your bladder becomes the star of the show, and your kidneys are working overtime like diligent night-shift employees.

The Emotional Acrobatics: Mood Swings Take the Stage

Now, don't be surprised if you're feeling like an emotional acrobat during the first trimester. Mood swings are like the opening act of this grand performance, showcasing the full range of human emotions. But do not worry, because the second trimester might just be the intermission you've been waiting for – a time of relative emotional stability.

Tender Milk Bar

Just think of them as your body's built-in milk bar, gearing up for the big opening night. Now, while they might be feeling a bit sensitive and achy due to all that increased blood flow, a supportive bra can be your superhero in this breast-related adventure.

And, oh yes, the color show – those nipples of yours might decide to embrace a few new darker shades – it will go back to normal, cross my heart and all that...

Hormonal Circus: Constipation Crashes the Party

Hold onto your hats, because that's not all the fun this hormonal circus has in store. Constipation's sneaking in too, like a surprise guest who overstays its welcome. Blame it on the progesterone parade – it's like the main act, but instead of rocking the stage, it's slowing down your digestive party.

Handy Tip: Load up on whole grains, fruits, and veggies – it's like sending constipation a stylish eviction notice. And don't forget to hydrate like a hydration superhero. Water is your sidekick, flushing away those unwelcome guests (poop...we are talking shit here) like the champ it is.

Shine bright like a disco ball

Your skin's joining the party with a "shine bright like a disco ball" mode. Thanks to the hormone extravaganza, your face might be producing more oil than a deep fryer at a carnival stand.

Oh, touché!

Pimple parade

It seems like the universe got wind of your nostalgic desires and decided to send you a blast from the past – a pimple parade to remind you of the good ol' days. So, thank you, universe, for this unexpected trip down memory lane.

Lesson learned!

Be careful what you wish for because the universe has a quirky sense of humor.

Things worth considering

- Did you decide on the doctor and the clinic? Not Yet? Time to do so ASAP!

- Embark on a closet expedition to round up the stretchiest, comfiest threads that you can find

- Give your sensitive bosom buddies some extra TLC by rocking a supportive bra even during nighttime hours.

- Keep the hydration train chugging along, munch on fiber-rich goodies

- Have your health superhero's number on speed dial for those "uh-oh" moments when your doctor's out for a coffee break.

- Stock up on folic acid and prenatal vitamins

- Take a peek at the list of symptoms that should definitely not be overlooked during this pregnancy stage. Just in case, it's good to know what to keep an eye out for and what to do if any of those worrisome signs decide to make an appearance.

Week 7 – 2nd month– 1st Trymester

Hold onto your excitement hats, because your tiny superstar is putting on a growth spurt that would make any blueberry envious!

Your baby

At seven weeks, your little embryo is strutting its stuff at a whopping 8 millimeters – talk about a tiny dynamo in action!

The inside scoop on the baby brain bonanza
While it'll keep growing well after the grand debut, the blueprint for this future genius is already laid out. And guess what? The construction crew is hard at work on the lungs and digestive system too – it's like a bustling baby construction site in there!

Artistry at its finest
Oh, but that's not all – your little Picasso is sculpting away on those adorable facial features, and those tiny hands are rockin' the paddle-palm look. It's like they're prepping to high-five you from the inside!

A mini-metro system of nourishment and waste removal
Let's not forget the star of the show – the umbilical cord! It's like your baby's lifeline, the ultimate nutrient highway connecting your world with theirs.

A little hint for the ultimate ear-gasm
If you're going for an ultrasound this week, you might just catch a symphony of joy – your baby's heartbeat! But if you're not on team ultrasound yet, no worries – patience is a virtue in this pregnancy adventure.

So, whether it's brain-building, lung launching, or hand high-fiving, your baby's got it all under control.

Your body

At seven weeks, your body's decided to throw a party like no other! It's like your hormones are the DJ, spinning tunes that make your emotions do the cha-cha. Meanwhile, your little peanut is growing faster than your love for late-night snacks – we're talking a mini-miracle in the making!

And let's not forget those surprise guests: the "pee-break posse" and the "snack attack squad." They're like your body's new BFFs, joining you on this wild ride. So, whether you're waltzing with mood swings, hosting a peanut-sized bash, or sneaking off for a snack safari, your body's in for the adventure of a lifetime – and trust me, it's a VIP invitation you won't want to miss!

Your doctor might have dropped the knowledge bomb about this sneaky infection called toxoplasmosis – it's like a germ ninja that loves to hang out in raw meat and cat poop.
Now, when it comes to kitty litter duty, it's time to delegate like a boss. Pass the scoop to a trusted household comrade – let them be the litter warrior while you focus on growing that amazing bun in the oven. It's like a chore swap, pregnancy style!

So, there you have it – your secret weapons against the toxo tag team: crispy well-done meat, soap and clean hands ballets, and a kitty litter deputy. As you navigate this germ-avoidance adventure, just remember, you've got this pregnancy game on lockdown, and toxoplasmosis doesn't stand a chance against you!

What symptomps you can expect in the week 7

Hold onto your pregnancy hats because those early symptoms you've been rockin' might just be sticking around like your very own fan club – and they might even be pulling out all the stops for a grand encore!
But don't let those pesky symptoms rain on your parade, because guess what? The second trimester is like the ultimate spotlight, ready to steal the show and dim those symptoms down.

Now, let's dive into the fabulous lineup for the seventh week – it's like your body's hosting its very own pregnancy variety show:

Morning Nausea & Pals

Yep, those morning waves might still be surfing in, and they might have invited some friends along. But don't worry, this gang tends to take a breather as the second-trimester steps in.

Bad news: Brace yourself, because those pesky symptoms might be hitting their peak performance right about now, bringing along their grumpy sidekick, the bad mood.

Good news: as the second trimester swoops in, many women find these troublemakers taking a backseat and bidding farewell.

Fatigue Fiesta

Your body's marathon of tiredness is still going strong. It's like the never-ending quest for the comfiest pillow fort. But hang tight, because soon enough, you'll be enjoying the perks of pregnancy energy. Progesterone levels continue to rise, and high levels of this hormone can cause drowsiness.

Pee Parade

That frequent restroom shuffle continues like your bladder's leading a parade route. But trust me, the second trimester might just be the golden ticket to fewer pit stops. But here's the twist: instead of pushing that hydration snooze button, embrace it with open arms – or shall we say, open water bottles? Hydrate like it's your full-time job, sipping that H2O like a boss.

Mood Swing Soiree

Emotions are still dancing to their own rhythm, like a wild carnival on an emotional roller coaster. But fear not, because the calm and collected second trimester is peeking around the corner.

Tender Tatas

Your bosom buddies might still be in the spotlight, getting all sensitive and achy. It's like they're rehearsing for their future milk star roles.

Super Smell Sensation

Your nose might be on high alert, detecting scents from a mile away. It's like you've got a superhero nose, ready to sniff out any scent caper.

Welcome to the saliva show

 Excessive saliva might be joining your pregnancy party, often waltzing in with the morning nausea crew. It's like a quirky cameo, but trust me, you're not the only leading lady in this script.

Food roulette, anyone?

Craving pickles and chocolate for dinner? Are eggs suddenly smelling like the worst party crasher? Blame it on the hormone orchestra – they're conducting a wild symphony of taste buds and scent sensors. And hey, if you're hankering for chalk or dirt, let your doctor know – they're the official taste testers of this pregnancy menu.

Drumroll, please... introducing the diarrhea dilemma!

Yep, your bathroom breaks might be getting extra special with a dash of diarrhea. But fear not, it's usually just a hormone-induced side act. Luckily, apple mousse, oatmeal, and bananas are here to save the day – they'll mop up the mess without leaving your body high and dry.

Cue the cramps!

Your expanding uterus is setting up shop and might be giving you some mild discomfort. Think of it as the warm-up for the big show. But if those cramps decide to go all diva on you, or if you sense anything more than just a crampy sensation, it's time to dial up your doctor for a VIP consultation.

Hey there, warrior of the womb! If those pregnancy symptoms have you feeling like you're in a mood funk, hang tight because the superhero second trimester is just a few weeks away.

Handy tip: If those mood swings are giving you a serious run for your joy, or if you're dealing with mental health concerns, don't hesitate to call in the professionals. Think of them as your emotional lifeguards, ready to help you ride those waves with grace. They've got the tools to make sure you're not battling those blues alone, so you can focus on rocking this pregnancy journey like the superhero you are. Remember, you're never alone on this adventure, and there's always a helping hand ready to guide you through the storm to the sunnier side.

Things to consider this week

Time to treat that skin like the precious canvas it is!
Acne might be staging a little takeover, but don't worry, you're the director of this skincare show. Grab your cleansing spotlight and give your complexion a thorough cleanse – it's like a glamorous red carpet treatment for your face. Blame it on the excessive sebum production causing those pesky clogs and pimples, but fear not, you've got this in the bag!

Nutrient Extravaganza: Prenatal Vitamins Take the Stage
And speaking of nutrients, roll out the red carpet for folic acid and its nutrient entourage by taking those prenatal vitamins like a pro. Your body's getting the VIP treatment, ensuring it's well-fed with all the good stuff.

Nourishment Party: Unveiling the Nutrient Entourage
Time to play nutrient detective and ensure you and your little sidekick are getting the ultimate nourishment party! But hey, let's keep those heartburn villains at bay – give spicy and fried foods the VIP boot from your menu. It's like an exclusive party where only the good stuff gets an invite.

Food Detective Mode
For all you veggie or vegan champs out there, it's time to plant-power up! Make sure your plate is rocking some fantastic plant-based proteins like grains and legumes – they're the VIP guests at your nutritional feast.

B12 Express: The Supplement Ticket for Non-Animal Product Passengers
If you're missing the B12 train (which only rolls through animal products town), consider grabbing a supplement ticket. It's like the express route to making sure your body's getting all the right notes in the nutrient symphony.

Hydration Headquarters
Hydrate like it's your full-time job, sipping that H2O like a boss.

And when in doubt, it's like having a direct line to the nutrition maestro – your doctor! They've got the secret sauce to balance out your dietary masterpiece.

Week 8 – 2nd month– 1st Trymester
Your baby

Hold onto your excitement hats, because that little toddler of yours is on the move and shaking things up!
They've already strutted quite a distance, and get ready, because their development is about to kick into high gear. This week, our pint-sized star is all about the raspberry-sized charm, measuring in at a cool 13 to 15 millimeters in parietal-limb length.

Oh, so cute...
Let's talk about those oh-so-cute fingers and toes – they're making their grand debut, complete with their very own mini membranes. And guess what? The hands are already showing off their bendy skills at the elbows and wrists. It's like a tiny acrobatic performance in the making!

Gender reveal?
But hold the gender reveal party for a bit, because even though the genitalia are in the works, the big "boy or girl" secret is still under wraps. It's like nature's surprise party, keeping you guessing for a little longer.

The internal superstar lineup – it's like a symphony of development behind the scenes. The gastrointestinal tract is gearing up for action, with the midgut loop making a temporary appearance in the umbilical cord's swanky space.
Yep, even at this stage, those intestines are hard at work, managing the body's metabolic show.

The plot twist!
In about a month's time, as the baby's abdomen gets roomier, those intestines will strut their stuff back into the abdominal cavity. It's like a choreographed dance, making sure everything's in the right place for the ultimate baby debut.

So there you have it, the raspberry-sized superstar and their grand development adventure, complete with acrobatic hands, secret gender mysteries, and mesmerizing internal performance.
Your little one is stealing the show, one tiny milestone at a time!

Congratulations, you've hit the eighth-week mark – and guess what, your clothes might be staging a little rebellion, but don't worry, you're still the star of this pregnancy show! Yep, those pants might be getting a tad snug, but let's focus on the bigger picture – the delightful (or maybe not-so-delightful) symphony of first-trimester sensations.

The ultimate silver lining

Amidst all the ups and downs, the highlight reel of your week is about to hit a high note. Get ready to turn up the volume, because the sweetest sound in the world is about to serenade your ears – your baby's heartbeat! It's like a melody of magic, making all those symptoms feel like a VIP concert ticket.

Baby bump watch

It's like anticipating the grand reveal in a movie plot. When will that adorable belly make its entrance? Well, buckle up, because it's like a personalized show for each mom-to-be. Not only do different pregnant mamas rock their own unique baby bump style, but even your future pregnancies might throw a plot twist in the mix.

But here's the ballpark figure: around the 13-week mark, you might notice your jeans exchanging secret glances with your baby bump. So, whether your clothes are going for a snug fit or your belly's embracing the limelight, know that your pregnancy journey is as unique and exciting as you are.

Possible symptoms for week 8

Hang in There Barfing Lady

Morning sickness – check! Still here. The good news is that the 2nd trimester is around the corner, and this symptom should ease off by then (fingers crossed).

Handy tip: Try to eat five/six small meals a day instead of three large ones.

Oops, It's Still Hanging Around

Diarrhea – yep! Still here as well. Drink up, eat well, and consult your doctor if it lasts for more than 24 hours.

Peeing Racehorse Style: Saddle Up for the Long Ride

Ah, the racehorse peeing – it's like your bladder's running its own marathon! Imagine your baby and uterus like roommates who are really into expansion – they're growing and spreading out, and your bladder's like, "Excuse me, coming through!" So, expect this tag-along to make appearances throughout the rest of the pregnancy, coming and going like a faithful friend.

Sensory Circus: Food and Smell Extravaganza for Your Nose

Get ready for the pregnancy adventure of the senses! Suddenly, foods and smells are putting on a circus act in your nose, like a smell-powered roller coaster that's making your tummy do loop-de-loops.

Spotting Canvas: Pregnancy's Artistic Intricacies

Now, let's talk spotting – it's like a pregnancy canvas, and a few artistic drops might make an appearance. But if that canvas starts resembling a masterpiece, with heavier bleeding or worry-inducing scenes, it's time to bring in the pregnancy art critic – aka your doctor.

Back Dance Party: Your Lower Back's Groovin' to a New Beat

Speaking of loops, your back might be doing a dance of its own – it's like a lower-back party zone as your muscles hustle to support your growing guest of honor, the uterus. Your body's shifting, your center of gravity's playing musical chairs, and those pregnancy hormones are on a mission to turn your pelvic joints into the ultimate limber yoga pros.

Sleep Saga: Pillow Hugs and Left-Side Lounging

Hormones, restroom rendezvous, and a general "pregnancy party" vibe might be keeping your sleep playlist on shuffle. If counting sheep isn't cutting it,

try a serenade of soothing music, dive into a book, or enjoy some warm milk

or a cozy shower before bedtime. And rumor has it, the left side's the cool kid for better blood circulation, so go ahead and give it a whirl. Plus, if a pillow

hug between your knees sounds like a sleepover perk, you're onto something comfy.

Things to consider this week

Smile Spa Day: Keeping Your Pearly Whites Happy
Schedule a date with your dentist, because they've got the personalized scoop on keeping your teeth and gums happy during this baby-making journey. It's like a dental spa day, complete with tips and tricks to keep your smile shining as bright as your pregnancy glow.

Stretchy Superhero Clothes: Your New BFFs in Comfort
Time to level up your closet game – those stretchy superhero clothes are your new BFFs, because your regular wardrobe might be getting a bit snug. It's like giving your outfits a comfy hug, and saying goodbye to tight pants – they're not invited to this party!

Breast Buddies: Growing Pals Deserve the Right Fit
And speaking of support, let's talk bras! Your breast buddies are growing, and they deserve the right fit. It's like giving them a cozy nest for their big adventure.

Workout Wonder: Keep That Active Flame Alive
Now, let's break a sweat – if you were a fitness aficionado before, don't worry, your favorite sports might still be on the menu. It's like keeping that active flame burning, but remember to have a little chat with your doctor to ensure your workout is pregnancy-approved. Safety first, superhero!

Baby Name Brainstorm: Creating the Name Treasure Chest
While the gender secrets are still locked away, why not kick-start the baby name brainstorm? It's like creating a name treasure chest, a gift for your future mini-me. Scribble those moniker marvels in your pregnancy diary – imagine your little one perusing your naming adventures with a smile a few years down the road.
And guess what? You've got months of name-play ahead, so don't stress, because you're the director of this naming masterpiece.

So, whether you're itching to share the news or savoring the secrecy, and whether you're scribbling names in your diary or setting the baby name stage, remember: you're crafting your own pregnancy narrative, full of twists, turns, and heartwarming moments that'll leave your heart and baby book brimming with joy.

Parent Party: Connect and Share the Baby Bonanza

Time to join the parent party – reach out and connect with fellow baby buddies who are sharing your pregnancy timeline! It's like a virtual baby bonanza through social media or even local parent support groups. Those parents nearby are a goldmine of wisdom and camaraderie – consider it a VIP ticket to the pregnancy advice and friendship club.

Doctor Casting Call: Choose Your Pregnancy Partner-in-Crime

It's time for your grand entrance at the gynecologist's office – your VIP ticket to excellent medical care. Choose your doctor like you're casting for the role of your pregnancy partner-in-crime. Look for a pro who's got that friendly sparkle, because they're the ones who'll be there for you through every pregnancy twist and turn.

The Grand Dilemma of Pregnancy Beans

Ah, the grand dilemma: to spill the pregnancy beans or to keep it under wraps? It's like a suspenseful plot twist with no right or wrong answer. Some couples throw a "Guess What?" party right away, while others play the waiting game until the first-trimester curtain call when the risk of spoilers (a.k.a. miscarriage) drops its dramatic entrance.

It is really up to you when you wish to share this amazing adventure with the outside world.

Cherry-Sized Celebrity: Your Tiny Wonder Upgraded!
Weighing in at a mighty 2 grams and measuring 15 to 18 mm, your little superstar is making quite the entrance.

Vanishing Tail Act: The Magic of Baby's Transformation
Say farewell to the tail – it's like a vanishing act from the earlier weeks. Your baby's transformation into a bona fide mini-human is in full swing, and that pink blob is giving way to a more defined little peck.

Facial Finesse Lessons: Nose, Eyelids, and Proportional Adorableness
Check out those facial finesse lessons – the nose and eyelids are stepping into the spotlight, and the head is rocking the "proportionally adorable" look with its larger-than-life presence. Oh, and those dainty toes are making their debut on the foot scene – it's like a mini foot fashion show.

Internal Construction Site
Internally, it's a bustling construction site – digestive and reproductive systems are under development, complete with some swanky intestines and potential future rock stars, aka testicles or ovaries.

And guess what? Your baby's got some groove now, flexing those newfound muscles. It's like a backstage dance party, and even though you won't feel those moves just yet, your little dancer is warming up for their grand performance in the second trimester.

A Cherry-Sized Sensation: Your Baby's Grand Entrance on the Stage of Development
Your pregnancy journey is writing its own masterpiece, and your baby is the star with moves that'll leave you in awe.

Get ready to cheer on the main act – you and your tiny cherry-sized marvel!

Ah, the boobie transformation saga continues!
In this ninth week of pregnancy, your lovely ladies are embracing their fullness and taking the stage as the main event. Thanks to those superstar mammary glands and some extra fatty tissue, they're all about that "fuller and heavier" vibe.

Hold onto your bra straps, because here's the plot twist – even though these boobie changes might feel like the star of the show now, they're actually just warming up for the grand performance. As your pregnancy tale unfolds, your breasts might keep growing, but the good news is that their newfound tenderness usually bows out as your body gets comfy with the hormone party.

Intricate Brush Strokes: Prominent Veins Tell the Story
Your breast masterpiece is getting an artistic touch, with more prominent veins, like intricate brush strokes telling the story of increased blood supply. Your nipples and areolas are getting in on the makeover too, with a potential shade change as hormones put their creative spin on things. It's like a little artistic flair in the midst of your amazing pregnancy canvas.

Pregnancy Play in the Sports Arena: Your Fitness Strategy
Time for a little pregnancy play in the sports arena! If you're a sports fanatic, consider it a game of strategy. If you're new to the field, it's your chance to join the fun and play safe.

Ladies, if you've got a love for sports, let's tweak that playbook. And if you're just stepping onto the court, no worries – it's never too late to start. Think of it like picking the perfect sporty outfit for your baby bump journey.

Tricky Jump Shots and Sudden Moves: Avoiding Joint Hurdles
Ready for some star moves? Walking, yoga tailor-made for expecting champs, and even a splashy swim or water aerobics session – these are your VIP passes to the pregnancy fitness club.

But watch out for those tricky jump shots and sudden moves – they might not be the best teammates for your joints. It's like giving your body a high-five and avoiding any joint hurdles.

But remember, before you embark on your sporty adventure, make a quick timeout and chat with your doc. They're the ultimate coaches to guide you to the winning fitness game plan. So, get ready to hit the field, find your fitness groove, and embrace your pregnancy journey with a winning spirit – you've got this, superstar!

Game of Hide and Seek: Your Baby Bump's Debut

And hey, don't worry if the belly's not playing peek-a-boo just yet. It's like a game of hide and seek, and for most MVP moms, those first pregnancy curves start showing up around the 13-week mark. Your baby bump's getting ready for its debut, and when it finally takes the stage, you'll be cheering on your own personal pregnancy superstar.

Possible symptoms for week 8

Here's the pregnancy playbook for your ninth week, starring some quirky symptoms:

Waistline expansion

Your belly's not the main act yet, but your jeans might be feeling a tad snug. Blame the hormones and a touch of bloating – it's like a sneaky costume change that comes with the pregnancy territory.

Rise and shine, or maybe not?

If the morning nausea hasn't crashed your pregnancy party yet, cheers to being part of the lucky crew. But if you find yourself playing patty-cake with pregnancy queasies, small and frequent meals plus a hydration station might be your golden ticket to feeling better.

Spotting

A sprinkle of spotting might pop up in this trimester's storyline. If it's more than just a few drops, ring up your doctor for a plot twist check.

Uterine charades

Your body's playing a dynamic game, and those mild uterine contractions might be joining the party. If they're going full-on drama or bringing in backup (hello, lower back pain), your doctor's the director to call.

Hungry much?
Your appetite's got its own storyline now, and it's craving the spotlight. Channel your inner snack wizard with some extra munchies – think fruit, cereal, or a yogurt cameo – because your pregnancy cravings are just getting started. And hey, don't forget the calorie count – it's like keeping your appetite superstar on track with a dash of pregnancy math.

Fatigue, the ultimate first-trimester superstar!
Thanks to the progesterone party, you might be ready to catch some z's at any moment. Embrace daytime siestas – they're like power-ups for your pregnancy journey, especially if your night-time sleep is playing hard to get.

Frequent potty breaks
Yep, the bathroom's your new BFF, thanks to your growing superstar and the bustling blood brigade. Your kidneys are working overtime, and your bladder's feeling the squeeze. Hydration's the name of the game, so drink up! Just sneak in a quick bathroom pit stop before you venture out – it's like a pre-mission bathroom briefing. And hey, if things start to burn or feel funky, signal your doctor – it's like a potential urinary SOS that needs a superhero check.

Cravings and "eww" moments
Your super-sniffer's in action, turning taste and scent into a rollercoaster ride. The stuff you once loved might suddenly seem like the villains of your palate, while new cravings could steal the spotlight.
Healthy cravings? Go for it! Just keep your culinary show balanced and diverse. But hey, if you're hankering for something wacky like dirt or chalk, that's a hotline to your doctor.

From "woohoo!" to "what just happened?"
That's the hormonal hocus-pocus of pregnancy at play. Share the drama with your support squad – chatting it out might just sprinkle some mood-boosting magic. And if those mood swings keep staging a takeover, don't hesitate to call in the doc for backup.

Well, hello there, surprise party on your face!
If acne decides to crash your pregnancy bash, blame it on those hormonal hiccups – they're the rowdy guests causing all the ruckus.
But hey, don't worry, this pimple party is just a temporary fiesta that'll pack up and leave after your baby's grand debut.

Wise words from the veteran parents in your squad
Before diving into the baby gear shopping spree, tap into their treasure
trove of advice. They'll happily spill the beans on must-haves, budget
savers, and the "do-we-really-need-that?" items, so you can stroll through
the layette aisle like a seasoned pro.

Time to curb the caffeine craving!
While coffee takes the spotlight, remember tea, sodas, and chocolate are
in on the act too. Keep the caffeine curtain at around 200 mg a day – that's
like sipping from a 350 ml coffee cup.

You've got this mama-bear

Your baby

Get ready to meet your strawberry-sized superstar!

At week 10, your little sidekick has gone from embryo to fetus at warp speed. The rounder, more human-like head is taking the stage, and inside, a symphony of organs is gearing up for action.

Teeth's tiny nuclei are even practicing their grand entrance in your baby's mouth.

Fingers and toes are stretching out, and those webbed membranes are fading like a backstage backdrop.

While the eyes, eyelids, and ears are still in their workshop phase, they've got some growing to do before they're red carpet ready.

So keep cheering on your berry-sized wonder – the show's just getting started!

Your body

Blood Flow Traffic Jam: Leg Veins Take Center Stage

As your pregnancy tale unfolds, your growing uterus can sometimes hog the limelight, causing a bit of a traffic jam for blood flow down below. When this curtain rises, leg veins might join the visible stars, with swelling and soreness in the spotlight.

Varicose veins might sneak into the scene, uninvited, but fret not – you're the director here. Keep those legs uncrossed, wave 'ta-ta' to excessive standing and sitting, and embrace the power of pregnancy-friendly compression tights (we are bringing sexy back, I know...).

Elevate those legs for a VIP blood flow experience, and if your doctor gives the nod, a touch of safe exercise can be a star in your daily show.

Fruity Transformation: From Pear to Grapefruit - Uterus Upgrade!

Inside your amazing 10-week pregnant body, a bustling orchestra of hormones and growth is in full swing. Organs are developing, blood flow is on the rise, and your uterus is expanding to accommodate your growing little star.

Your uterus is on a fruity journey, upgrading from pear to grapefruit status! It's all part of the marvelous transformation happening within you. Keep embracing the changes and soon you'll be sporting a full-on fruit basket!

Sneak Peek into the Fabulous Future: Stretchy Attire Upgrade

Your baby bump might not be stealing the spotlight just yet (although some bump stars do debut early!), so your regular wardrobe still has its moment. But hey, a stretchy attire upgrade? Time to give your closet a sneak peek into the fabulous future!

What's new (or still here) in week 10?

Barf-vaganza

Time for a scoop of news: the "barfing party" might still be in full swing. But here comes the glimmer of hope – the second trimester is just around the corner, and it often brings relief from the nausea saga.

Now, here's the bonus round: some moms-to-be get an extra ticket to the wild ride known as "hyperemesis gravidarum" – a fancy name for super intense pregnancy vomiting. If you think you might be starring in this show, don't hesitate to chat up your doc – they've got the backstage pass to help you out.

Power Nap Craving: Answer Like a Pro

Embrace the power nap craving! Blame it on the progesterone party in your body – those energy levels might be playing hide and seek. So if a nap calls your name, answer it like a pro. You're not just napping, you're recharging for the epic journey ahead – so snooze away, my dear mama-to-be.

The Drama of the Oblique Ligament Plot

These pelvic superheroes, the obturator ligaments, are on a mission to support your growing uterus. So, here's the deal: if you're feeling a little discomfort or even a touch of "ouch" on one or both sides, blame it on the ligament divas. Sometimes they throw a tantrum when you switch positions in bed or hit the exercise mat too hard. The good news is, that gentle stretches and exercises can help to manage the pain. But if they decide to stay on, or a fever gatecrashes the party, it's your cue to dial your doc – they've got the script for your relief!

Partner's Dragon Wake-Up Call: Hormonal Escape Tactics

Hormones are rocking the spotlight at 10 weeks, staging emotional roller coasters that even the wildest theme parks would applaud. And if your partner's suddenly sprinting in the opposite direction at home, well, let's be real – it's all about avoiding that dragon wake-up call.

Discharge Disclosure: Colorless Flow, Strange Vibes Alert!

All right, let's talk discharge – yeah, the less glamorous part of the pregnancy journey. So, here's the scoop: that down-there flow might amp up a bit due to all the extra blood circulation and those hormone parties happening down below. Now, normal discharge should be colorless or milky white, with hardly any scent, and chilling on the low-down. But if it starts flashing unusual colors or giving off strange vibes (itching, weird smells, or unexpected bleeding), it's time to signal your doctor. Remember, it's all about keeping things smooth & odor-free down there!

The Headache Hustle: Ice Packs and Headlining Acts

Pregnancy can throw a curveball at your noggin sometimes. If you find yourself in a head-spinning showdown, retreat to a dimly lit room – it's your headache sanctuary. And here's the cool trick: grab an ice pack, let it work its magic on your head or neck, and watch the pain do a disappearing act. But, if the headache turns into a marathon runner or feels like a rock concert gone wrong, don't be shy – give your doctor a ring for the ultimate headlining act!

Weight Gain Cool Down: No Waistband Panic... Yet!

No need to panic about the waistband – yet! – as your weight gain might be playing it cool and be there but only on a minimal side. If first-trimester tummy turbulence had you doing the "up and down" dance with your scale, don't stress. We've got the backstage scoop on weight gain during pregnancy, and your doctor's ready to chime in with their wisdom.

Acne's Party Crash: Hang Tight, Mama!

Acne, you sly little troublemaker, you've decided to crash the pregnancy party. The good news? This skin thingy should wrap up once the baby makes their grand entrance.

Unveiling Pregnancy's Plot Twists

As you embark on this chapter of your pregnancy adventure, it's time for those debut gynecological and general check-ups. A round of laboratory tests takes the stage, aiming to uncover any potential infections, decode your blood type and Rh factor, and even seek out those elusive immune antibodies in your blood plasma. It's a plot twist you didn't see coming, but fear not – your healthcare team has got the script down to a science!

All Aboard the Decaf Train!

Time to bid farewell to the coffee locomotive (no judgment here, I've had my own tussle with coffee-induced acrobatics, but I kept sipping).

The Honeymoon Stage Getaway

Picture this: a getaway during your "honeymoon stage" of pregnancy – a time when your morning barfing takes a break (fingers crossed), your hormonal rollercoaster transforms you from a dragon to a friendly lizard, and you can still sneak a peek at those toes (they're not forgotten!).

So, mama-to-be, treat yourself to some well-deserved R&R because, trust me, you'll appreciate that relaxing escape more than a chocolate stash hidden from craving monsters!

Week 11 of the baby-making marathon, and guess what? Our star player is now rocking the Brussels sprout look. Yep, about 5 centimeters of pure potential, weighing in at a whopping 9 grams. It's like having a pocket-sized miracle!

This week is like a grand makeover episode for our tiny protagonist. From that big ol' noggin to the tiniest toothbud, everything's on the move and shaking.

Facial features? Check.

Ears on the move? You bet.

And those peepers? Well, they're keeping their "closed for now" sign-up – eyelids shut!

Oh, and let's not forget the classified bits – the baby's forming its private parts, but nope, the doctor's still got a "Wait, is it a boy or girl?" expression. And here's the funny part – that head? It's like a little alien, taking up half the space. But don't worry, the rest of the gang (torso and limbs) are queuing up for growth spurts soon.

With all this turbocharging growth, your tiny human's demanding more grub – more red blood cells and a plumper placenta are kicking in to keep up with the demand.

Go, mini-human, go!

Your body

What's cookin', good lookin'?"
Hey there, nose on high alert or are we into some unconventional munchies? Seriously, this symptom is like something Sherlock Holmes would chuckle at. Get this, they say 50 to 90 percent of expecting moms dive into offbeat flavors during pregnancy. You are in good company, my dear...

No one-size-fits-all answer for this quirk

On one hand, they say your inner kitchen squad knows what your body craves, so they're like, "Here, have some of this!" On the other hand, it could be those hormones in the kitchen just messing with the whole taste bud orchestra. So, as long as your culinary expeditions stay within the "healthy and balanced pregnancy diet" territory, feast away!

Cautionary munchin' tale

If your cravings start veering into uncharted culinary territory – like clay or dirt, seriously? – it's time to ring up your doctor. Because even though chefs play around, experimenting with inedible stuff might not be your finest dish.

Fun part – what could be bugging you this week?

Booby Balloon Party!

Your breasts might be throwing a little bash – they're likely puffing up a bit and, brace yourself, they might continue their inflation journey as your pregnancy keeps trucking. Oh, and be ready for some serious lifting – during pregnancy, your breasts might decide to weigh more than a kilogram (over 2,2 pounds!) extra compared to your pre-pregnancy era.

Vaginal discharge? Yeah, still there.

Don't worry, though – it's a totally normal part of the pregnancy package. As long as it's not stinky and comes in shades of clear or white, it's all good. But, if you spot anything like blood, feel itchiness, or catch a whiff of something funky, it's "Hello, Doctor!" time to make sure everything's on track.

Leg Drama, Nighttime Edition

Brace yourself for the leg cramp theatrics during this pregnancy ride, especially when the moon's out. Some good ol' stretching and leg-focused exercises can be your backstage pass to relief. And here's a twist – these cramps might even be yelling for more calcium and magnesium in your diet. Oh, and don't forget to hydrate like a champ, just to keep things running smoothly.

Good ol' morning barf

Sorry, no better news here but keep in mind that this discomfort often takes its leave when the second trimester rolls in. So, you're on the home stretch now, really!

Fatigue Fiesta.

It's like your body went on a progesterone parade, and drowsiness is leading the march. And let's be real, it picks the least convenient moments to strike. Nighttime gets its own dose of disruption – bathroom breaks, leg cramps surprise parties, and even heartburn might crash the scene. But fear not, soldier! Boot caffeine out of the party and invite relaxation exercises instead. Combat those pregnancy yawns – you can do it!

Hormonal rollercoaster

Keep stress at bay and make sure you're getting enough iron – it's like a secret weapon against the emotional tornado. Want more tools in your arsenal? Try yoga, meditation, or serenading yourself with soothing music. And hey, if these mood swings turn into full-blown daily drama, don't hesitate to ask your doctor for some mood-enhancing advice. Your family will silently thank you.

The Abdominal Artistry

You might catch a glimpse of a unique streak on your abdomen – it's like a dark stripe showing up for the party. They call it the "linea negra" or black line, and it's like your body's personal artwork inspired by hormonal changes.
Pretty cool, right? And don't worry if it seems to steal the spotlight; it's just a temporary gig. Once the baby's out, the black line's making its exit too, stage left!

Some things to consider

Hey, Dads!

Pops-to-be, you might wanna peek into the realm of paternity leave and parental perks. Your workplace or even government programs might have some surprises in store. Time to dive into that paperwork!

The Birthplace Contemplation

Where's your little one going to make their grand entrance? You don't need to whip out the decision dice yet, but it's a great time for some birthplace brainstorming. Seek advice from your doc or midwife, and tap into the treasure trove of experiences from other local moms.

Vitamin C Superhero

Your baby-building journey craves around 80-85 milligrams of vitamin C daily. It's like the power boost for your baby's growth, from new cells to strong bones and teeth. So, throw some tangy oranges and zesty citrus fruits, along with strawberries, tomatoes, and even broccoli, into your culinary mix. It's like a tasty dose of vitamin C goodness.

Share the Love

Baby on board? Time to think about spreading the good news! Most parents-to-be spill the beans to family, friends, and work buddies either at the end of the first trimester or the beginning of the second. It's like launching your own happy news campaign!

Genetic Testing 101

Time for a genetic test pop quiz! What's recommended for your unique pregnancy? Need to chat about chorionic villus biopsy or nuchal translucency ultrasound? Your pregnancy conductor (aka your doctor) has all the deets.

Rhymes with Antibodies

Check the compatibility of your blood with your baby's by testing for anti-Rh antibodies. Oh, and partners, you might be in for the test too.

Tag, you're both it!

Passion Fruit-sized Wonder: Week 12 Pregnancy Update!
Welcome to the twelfth week of pregnancy, where your growing bundle of joy is now the size of a passion fruit – cute, right? We're talking about a parietal and sitting length of around 6.3 centimeters and a weight of approximately 14 grams.

Goodbye First Trimester: Crafting Body Parts and Organ Secrets
Guess what? You're on the brink of waving goodbye to the first trimester! But don't think your baby's been lounging around all this time. Nope, by the end of this week, your little superstar will have crafted a full house of body parts and organs, including the secret sex organs. Sneaky, right?

The Heartbeat Symphony: Catching a Doppler Serenade
That adorable heartbeat is likely vibing away, and if you're lucky enough to have a doctor's appointment lined up, you might just catch a listen on a Doppler machine. Music to your ears, right?

I have an eye on you!
Speaking of eyes, your baby's got the peepers all sorted out. Their eyelids are in the building – kind of fused together for now, but they'll open up and become more sociable by the end of the second trimester.

Arms vs. Legs: Baby's Growth Showdown
Little Mr. or Miss has got some growing priorities too. Those hands are a tad more advanced than the feet right now, and the arms are stealing the length show from the legs. Oh, and don't miss the tiny nail beds throwing a nail party on those fingers and toes. These nails are like the life of the party, growing right up to the grand finale – birth!

Building a Masterpiece: Baby's Construction Zone
And guess what? Your baby's making moves! But hold your horses, Mama, you'll start feeling those delightful kicks in a few more weeks.
Meanwhile, on the inside, it's like a full-blown construction zone – organs, muscles, and all things baby are coming together like a masterpiece.
Time to sit back, marvel at the miracle, and prepare for the next exciting chapters!

The Gender Secret: Keeping the Excitement Alive

Hang in there! The gender secret's still under wraps, nestled snugly beneath your heart. Patience is the name of the game. The big reveal will come your way soon, so stay excited and keep those guessing games alive!

Your body

Morning Sickness Farewell: Appetite Takes the Stage!

Say goodbye to the morning sickness marathon – your appetite might just stage a triumphant comeback! But don't be surprised if it comes back with a vengeance.

Now, here's the culinary scoop: Balancing quantity and quality is key. Experts give a thumbs-up to adding around 300 extra calories to your daily menu during pregnancy. For a personalized roadmap, your doctor's the guru to consult, so don't hesitate to ask for some sage advice on a nourishing pregnancy diet.

Protein pals, this one's for you!

Whether you're into meats, fish, or plant-based goodness, protein is your buddy. Load up on veggies and fruits like they're going out of style – they're like a treasure trove of vitamins and minerals. And hey, don't forget the calcium crew: low-fat dairy, beans, nuts, and tofu. These buddies are your calcium superheroes!

Belly Business: Embracing the Unique Canvas of Pregnancy Curves

Staring at your midsection and doing the comparison dance? Hold up! Each pregnancy is like a unique masterpiece, and your belly's size is painted with a unique brush. It's like your physique, pre-pregnancy weight, whether this is your first rodeo, and even if it's a single or multiple-baby affair – all these factors get their creative say. So, whether your belly's rocking a little roundness or not, don't sweat it. Those pregnancy curves are like stealthy artists – they'll make their debut right on time!

Gum Gripe

Pregnancy's got some surprises, and one of them might be those sensitive gums saying, "Hey, we're here too!" Blood volume's doing a happy dance, and hormones are throwing a party – all of which might lead to swollen and tender gums. Maybe you've even noticed a bit of bleeding while you brush or floss. Fret not, this is a classic pregnancy ensemble, and chances are there's no need to sound the alarm bells. Keep up with your oral hygiene game – regular brushing and flossing are the MVPs. If you're in doubt, give your dentist a call to confirm that all's well.

Pro tip: Soft-bristled toothbrushes and a saltwater rinse (just dissolve a teaspoon of salt in a cup of warm water) can be your gum-soothing allies.

Feeling like the room's doing a spin?

It's all in the name of pregnancy! Blood vessels are doing their stretch routine, and hormones are like a rollercoaster ride. Result? Dizziness and momentary weakness might decide to pop by. Stay comfy in loose clothes, keep that hydration train chugging along, snack smartly, and avoid superhero-style standing marathons.
Oh, and the grand finale? No sudden position switches – rise slowly and gracefully. Now, if this dizzy drama's a persistent guest or comes with buddies like abdominal pain or vaginal bleeding, that's the cue to ring up your doctor for some expert advice.

Smell Superhero Mode

Hold onto your nose – your super sniffer might be in overdrive! That food aroma intensifies, and if it's becoming a bit much, switch to cooler or room-temperature eats. Oh, and having a fan on duty while cooking? Genius move. And hey, delegate the trash duty to someone else in the house, just for the moment. Your sensitive nose will thank you.

Gassy Galaxy

Hormones are playing games with your digestive system, and that can lead to some, well, interesting sounds and sensations. Eating in slow-mo might be your new jam. It helps to not swallow air along with your food, which can defuse the bloating bomb and make you feel way more comfortable.

Spotted Drama

If you spot some spotting (more than just a hint of light spotting, like after some bedroom action) around the 12-week mark, don't hit the panic button. But do dial up your doctor – especially if there's bleeding that's accompanied by cramps. It's like a safety check to ensure that everything's cruising smoothly in the baby-making journey.

Worth considering

Teeth Checkup To-Do

Time to give those pearly whites some attention. Schedule that dental check-up – keeping your oral health in tip-top shape is all part of the pregnancy superhero package.

Parenting Prep 101

Prenatal classes and birthing schools, anyone? Researching local options is like prepping for the ultimate adventure. Get some help from your doc or midwife, figure out when these classes kick off, and jot down the application deadlines. Education is the name of the parenting game!

Boss Talk Time

Pondering the right moment to give your boss the baby news? It's like a strategic move in the work chess game. Decide when feels right for you, and remember, you've got this!

Hey there, future pelvic floor champ!

Time to give those Kegel muscles a little workout. These unsung heroes support your uterus and bladder and even come with a bonus – preventing incontinence during pregnancy and post-baby time.
Here's the drill: Flex those pelvic floor muscles like you're stopping the flow of urine or holding back some gas. Squeeze and hold for a few seconds, then release. Start small with three sets of twenty reps daily. As those muscles beef up, feel free to amp up the repetitions and hold time.
Your pelvic floor will be like, "Thanks for the love!"

Week 13: It's Peachy!

You're in the 13th week of this incredible pregnancy journey, and guess what? Your precious little tenant in the belly is now rocking the size of a juicy plum or a dainty peach! Imagine that – your belly is hosting a mini fruit party!

Buzzing Workshop: Baby's Organ Orchestra

Now, I know it's like trying to guess the plot of a movie you've only seen the trailer for, but inside that cozy baby HQ of yours, things are buzzing. Think of it as a bustling workshop where tiny organs have set up shop and are already in full swing. It's like your baby's personal orchestra has started playing its first notes!

Housing upgrade

The superstar's kidneys have taken on a new gig – they're producing little squirts of baby urine, which gets a one-way ticket to the amniotic fluid swimming pool.

Meanwhile, the spleen is on duty, sifting through blood and giving the nod of approval to those red blood cells that carry the all-important oxygen. It's like having a mini quality control manager right there!

And hey, talk about a housing upgrade! The baby's intestines, which were sort of chilling near the belly button, are moving into the fancy new digs in the abdominal neighborhood. There's ample space, and they're settling in like they own the place.

Oh, and let's not forget those mini-construction projects! Some of the bony structures, including the head honcho skull, are getting their act together and getting harder by the day. Baby's building a strong foundation right from the start.

Tuning Up the Vocal Cord Orchestra: Future Coos and Giggles on the Way!
But wait, there's more! Your little munchkin might not be auditioning for 'The Voice' just yet, but guess what? The vocal cord orchestra is tuning up! You won't hear the oohs and ahhs until later, but those vocal cords are getting warmed up for the future cutest coos and giggles.

So, even though you can't exactly get a backstage pass to the action, know that there's a full-on party happening in there. Your baby's turning every week into a new adventure, and you're the best host this party could ask for!

Your body

Second Trimester: The "Honeymoon" Phase of Pregnancy
Congratulations, you've officially stepped into the second trimester of this amazing baby-making adventure! Many moms-to-be affectionately dub this phase the "honeymoon" of pregnancy – and no, it's not about romantic getaways with your cravings. It's all about waving goodbye to those pesky first-trimester woes.

Energizer Bunny Mode: Goodbye Fatigue, Nausea, and Frequent Bathroom Trips!
Farewell, fatigue! Adios, nausea! And hey there, not-so-frequent bathroom trips! They're all taking a well-deserved vacation right about now. But hold on, because that's not all – brace yourself for an energy boost that might just make you want to dance the cha-cha in your living room!

Imagine this trimester as a full-on switch in your body's production. It's like someone flipped a magical energy lever, and suddenly, you're the Energizer Bunny ready to take on the world.

The Placenta's Star Power: Commanding Your Blood Supply
Your blood supply and flow are now under the expert command of the placenta, which is growing as impressively as a superhero's cape in a comic book.

By the time your little bundle of joy makes its grand entrance, that placenta will be strutting the stage at about 700 grams – talk about some serious star power!

Uterine Fundus Height Test: Sizing Up Your Baby's Cozy Abode
As your pregnancy journey unfolds, your trusty doc will be keeping an eye on things. They'll whip out their measurement tape and perform the uterine fundus height test, basically measuring the distance from your pubic bone to the top of your ever-expanding uterus. It's like a size check for your baby's cozy abode. This little trick helps your doc figure out how far along you are and if your baby's hitting those development milestones like a champ.

Breast Tenderness: That One Friend Who Keeps Popping In
Now, let's talk about those lovely ladies up front – yep, your breasts. While you're soaking up the second-trimester sunshine, they might still be doing their own thing, giving you a friendly reminder of their presence. Just like that one friend who pops in and out unexpectedly, breast tenderness might come and go, leaving you wondering if they've got some secret agenda.

Pregnancy Amnesia: When Your Brain Adds Whimsy to the Adventure
If your dreams have suddenly transformed into Hollywood blockbuster productions or if you find yourself in a constant tug-of-war with your focus, don't worry. You're not on a solo journey to the land of peculiarities. "Pregnancy amnesia" is a card-carrying member of the pregnancy symptom club! It's like your brain's way of saying, "Hey, let's add a touch of whimsy to this adventure."

How you might feel in week 13

Ah, the thirteenth week of this amazing journey – you're officially in the sweet spot of pregnancy! Here's the scoop on some of the delightful and, let's say, interesting things you might be experiencing:

Bathroom Breaks and Discharge: The VIP Bouncer for Your Lady Parts
First up, the bathroom buddies. You might notice that your bathroom breaks are like clockwork, and that milky-white discharge making its entrance. Surprise! That discharge might not be the guest you expected, but it's like the VIP bouncer for your lady parts. It's there to keep everything protected and happy, defending against unwanted guests like infection and irritation. If it's causing a bit of a scene, don't worry – think of sanitary pads as your VIP pass to comfort.

Heartburn: The Uninvited Guest of Pregnancy

Oh, we've got heartburn. It's like an uninvited guest that just won't leave, and it might even RSVP for the entire pregnancy. You see, as your baby sets up shop and shifts around like a tiny acrobat, your stomach starts feeling a bit crowded. Blame it on the ever-growing uterus and its pressure antics.

But wait, there's more to the story – those sneaky pregnancy hormones decide to throw a curveball. They convince the muscles on top of your stomach to take a chill pill, allowing stomach acid to play the part of the party crasher in your esophagus. Cue the heartburn, our not-so-welcome friend.

Embrace Good Posture and Avoid Trigger Foods

Now, picture this: You've had a satisfying meal, and the urge to lie down and enjoy a post-feast siesta is oh-so-tempting. But hold on to your reclining chairs! Lying down can actually give heartburn the spotlight it's been craving. The good news? Your trusted allies are sitting up straight and avoiding heartburn's favorite treats – think chocolate, citrus fruits, and the spicy stuff. So, skip the melodramatic lie-down scenes and embrace the proud posture of
a queen.

Pregnancy and Intimacy: The Roller Coaster of Desire

Now, let's talk about the sizzle in the bedroom. Pregnancy is like a roller coaster for your desire meter. Sometimes it's on the wild side, and other times it's more chill. But guess what? That's totally normal! If you and your partner are feeling the groove and there are no red flags from your doctor, go ahead and have some fun – the baby's got a cushy setup in your personal baby castle (your uterus and amniotic sac are the best bodyguards in town).

But hey, if you've got questions swirling around your mind like confetti, your doctor's your go-to confidante. If a previous pregnancy felt like it ended on a sour note or your current one has a few curveballs, they might recommend a rain check on the intimate scenes – it's all about keeping things cozy and safe.

Constipation: Blame It on Hormones and Recruit Your Fiber Superheroes

Yes, those hormones are at it again! Progesterone and estrogen, the stars of the pregnancy show, have some side gigs, including slowing down your digestive system.

Think of it as a gentle reminder that your body is nurturing new life. Unfortunately, the sluggish system can lead to some roadblocks in the plumbing department. But don't worry, we're not leaving you stranded without a plan. It's time to recruit your fiber superheroes – fruits, veggies, and whole-grain foods. They're like the action heroes that swoop in and save the day by improving your bowel function. And let's not forget the hydration army – water is your trusty sidekick in this battle against constipation.

Oh, and here's a little secret weapon: dried prune juice. It might sound a bit old-school, but it's a tried-and-true remedy. And hey, even a bit of regular exercise joins the team to keep things moving smoothly.

The magical journey of colostrum: A Sneak Peek of What's to Come
Picture this: You're going about your day, and suddenly there's a little surprise on your shirt. No worries, though – it's just colostrum making its grand entrance.
Colostrum, the superhero version of breast milk, is like the VIP guest who arrives before the big party. It's thick, it's yellow, and it's packed with all sorts of goodies to welcome your little one to the world. It's like a nutritious pre-game for your baby's tummy.

Now, before you grab a panic button, know that this colostrum cameo is completely normal. Your body's just getting ready to be the world's best milk bar once your baby makes their debut. But hey, if you're not exactly thrilled about this unexpected leaky situation, consider it a chance to embrace your inner fashionista. Grab some trusty disposable or cotton breast pads – they're like the style guardians of your shirt. Just make sure they're made of natural materials to keep things comfortable and cozy.

Things to consider

When to Share the Pregnancy News with Family and Friends
The second trimester is like the grand stage for your big reveal. You see, as you step into this trimester, the chances of any unwanted plot twists like miscarriage significantly decrease.
But here's the deal – the spotlight's on you, and the decision to spill the beans is totally in your hands.

Pregnancy and Work: Timing the Big Announcement and Maternity Leave

Now, speaking of beans, let's talk business beans. If you're a working
wonder, it's time to put on your planning hat. When to share the baby
news with your employer is a bit like timing a perfectly baked soufflé –
it's gotta be just right. Once you've let the cat out of the bag, it's a stellar
move to keep your boss and colleagues in the loop about your impending
plans. That way, they can get the party hats ready for your maternity
leave.

Planning for Baby's Arrival: Nannies, Facilities, and Parental Benefits

If work's still in the picture, here's a key puzzle piece: maternity leave.
It's like a well-deserved break for you to soak in those baby cuddles. But
hey, it's also good to know the fine print. How many months of paid
maternity leave are you entitled to? When can you hit the pause button?
And here's the cherry on top – see if your employer serves up extra
parental benefits. It's like discovering a bonus level in the game of life.

Now, let's switch lanes to the baby care highway. Thinking about what's
next after the baby arrives? Planning ahead is like having a road map for
the journey. Friends can be like treasure troves of recommendations for
trusted nannies or top-notch facilities. It's like getting the inside scoop
on the best spots in town.

Exercise During Pregnancy: Keep Up Your Fitness Routine

And let's not forget about those super-powered workouts! If you're
already strutting your stuff in the fitness arena, keep up the
awesomeness. But if you're thinking of dipping your toes into the exercise
pool for the first time, a chat with your doc is like consulting with a wise
oracle. Walking, swimming, and even a little yoga can be your trusty
companions on this journey. Your muscles will be singing your praises,
especially when the baby arrives and you're dealing with the ultimate tag
team challenge.

Exercise Safety: Ab Workouts and Pelvic Floor Health

Oh, and a heads-up about those ab workouts – if your routine included
some crunches in the supine position, it's time for a little switcheroo.
When the uterus starts pulling a growth spurt, being on your back can
create some traffic jams for your blood flow. So, chat with your doc about
safe swaps to keep those muscles happy and the baby on board with the
adventure.

Let's dive into the realm of exercise even further – this time, we're talking about the unsung heroes: your pelvic floor muscles. These little champs play a big role in your journey. Imagine them as the backbone of bladder control and the ultimate support team for your pelvic organs – think bladder, uterus, small intestine, and rectum. Strengthening these muscles can be your secret weapon for a smoother ride.

Strengthening Your Pelvic Floor: The Importance of Kegel Exercises

Enter the stage: Kegel exercises! It's like a secret handshake for your pelvic floor. Here's the deal – squeeze and release those muscles down there, and you're on your way to pelvic power. You've got options: go for the long game with three solid squeezes followed by three releases, or opt for the quickfire version with multiple rapid contractions and relaxations. It's like your pelvic muscles are doing their own mini-workout routine.

Check with your doc

1. **Pelvic Pain Clarification:** Sometimes pelvic discomfort might make you wonder if everything's okay. Ask your doctor about the possible cause of the pain – could it be related to the round ligament stretching due to your growing uterus? Understanding the reasons behind it can provide some reassurance.

2. **Weight Gain Guidance:** Weight gain is part and parcel of pregnancy, but it's always a good idea to discuss it with your doctor. They can let you know if your current weight gain aligns with the healthy range and give you advice on any necessary adjustments.

3. **Chorionic Villus Biopsy:** If there's any recommendation for a chorionic villus biopsy, you should definitely discuss this with your doctor. This test is sometimes done to detect genetic conditions in the baby. Your doctor can explain the procedure, its benefits, and potential risks based on your medical history.

4. **Twin Pregnancy Considerations:** If you're expecting twins, there are specific things to consider. Your doctor can guide you on nutrition, prenatal care, potential complications, and what to expect during a twin pregnancy. They'll tailor their advice to your unique situation.

Remember, your doctor is your go-to source for accurate and personalized information. It's all about creating a safe and healthy environment for both you and your baby.

Your baby

Tiny Tots and Nectarines: A Comedy in 42 Grams

At 14 weeks of pregnancy, your baby is growing and developing rapidly, resembling the size of a nectarine. The average weight of your little one is around 42 grams, and their parietal-peripheral length (CRL) measures about 9 centimeters.

Thick Skin and Tiny Toes: A Baby's Guide to Inner Beauty

Your baby is becoming quite active this week, with their eyeballs beginning to move, and those tiny arms and legs starting to bend and flex. These movements are crucial as they practice bringing their hands to their mouth.

As the senses of smell and taste develop, your baby's skin is also thickening. While the suspense of whether your baby will have a full head of hair will continue until birth, the groundwork for hair growth is being laid beneath the skin's surface.

The Gender Mystery: Boy or Girl, the Suspense Unfolds!

With every passing week, your baby's appearance becomes more defined, bringing them closer to the little person you'll meet on the magical day of their arrival. While the genitals are fully developed, it might still be a bit early to determine the gender of your baby. The excitement of whether it's a boy or a girl will unfold in due time.

Your body

Welcome to the second trimester of your pregnancy!

This is the phase where your pregnancy belly begins to make its appearance, although the timing can vary for each mom-to-be. Keep in mind that every pregnancy journey is unique, so whether your curves show up a bit earlier or later, it's all normal. And if your pregnancy belly isn't quite showing yet, that's completely okay too! You might start noticing that your jeans are fitting a bit snugger, which is a charming reminder of the incredible changes happening within.

During your prenatal checkups, your doctor will start keeping track of the size of your abdomen and uterus. They'll measure the distance from your pubic bone to the top of your uterus to monitor your baby's growth. This measurement reflects how your uterus is expanding upwards to accommodate your growing baby since the moment of conception. It's a helpful way for your doctor to ensure that everything is progressing as it should. So, embrace the changes in your belly and the exciting journey ahead!

Welcome to the "honeymoon" phase of pregnancy!
This is the time when many moms-to-be experience a welcome relief from some of the more challenging symptoms of the first trimester, and a few positive changes often come their way.

Here are a couple of the most common perks you might enjoy:
1.   **Surge of Energy:** It's like a burst of sunshine after the storm. Many moms find that their energy levels pick up during the second trimester. If you're one of them, it's a refreshing change from the fatigue that might have been weighing you down in the first few months. As you progress further, especially into the third trimester, you might notice your energy tapering off a bit. So, make the most of this energetic phase to tackle important tasks.
2.   **Gorgeous Hair:** Yes, you read that right! Pregnancy can actually do wonders for your hair. For many women, hair becomes thicker and grows a bit faster than usual. It's one of those delightful changes that might put a smile on your face as you watch your locks flourish.

What you might expect in week 14

Here are a couple of experiences you might have during the 14th week of your pregnancy journey:

The Great Appetite Comeback: Pregnancy's Culinary Adventure
Farewell, persistent nausea! With that gone, you might find your appetite making a triumphant return. Embrace the newfound freedom from queasiness and indulge in some hearty eating.

Just remember to keep it balanced and nutritious. If your pre-pregnancy weight was in the healthy range (check your BMI if it falls between 18.5 and 24.9), you'll need to add around 300 extra calories to your daily intake (double that if you're expecting twins).

Pregnancy Rhinitis: When Your Nose Takes the Piss

Feeling like your nose is in perpetual "runny mode"? It's not uncommon during pregnancy. Blame it on the hormone progesterone, which can cause the blood vessels in your nasal passages to expand, leading to that stuffy feeling. It's even got a fancy name - pregnancy rhinitis. While there's no magic cure, staying hydrated can help you feel a bit better.
You might also find relief from using a humidifier or dabbing a little Vaseline around your nostrils to prevent dryness. Rinsing your nose with a saline solution might provide some relief too.

Leaking Secrets: Colostrum - The Baby's Sneak Peek

Don't be surprised if you notice a thick, yellowish fluid leaking from your breasts. This is colostrum, a special substance that's a nutritional powerhouse for your baby during the first few days after birth (we have this mentioned in previous weeks).
It's like a power-packed prelude to the milk that will come in later. While it might catch you off guard, rest assured that it's completely normal. You can use cotton breast pads to manage the leakage and stay comfortable.

Calf Cramps: The Nighttime Tango of the Second Trimester

While you're cruising through the second trimester, watch out for those pesky calf cramps that might decide to make an appearance, especially at night. But fear not, there are ways to give them the slip. Try some gentle stretching exercises before you hit the sheets, and make sure you're staying hydrated throughout the day. If the cramps still try to steal the show, give them a run for their money by giving your calf muscles a soothing massage or hopping into a warm bath or shower. It's all about keeping those cramps in check!

Remember, every pregnancy adventure comes with its quirks and surprises. Stay curious and take care of yourself, superstar!

Germs, beware!
Pregnancy's got the immune system doing the cha-cha. Catching a cold or flu might be trickier, so arm yourself with a flu shot and keep up with those
hand-washing heroics. And if a friend's sneezing like a confetti cannon, maybe give 'em a virtual high-five for now.

Time for a toothy adventure!
Schedule a date with the dentist for a smile check-up and cleaning. Pregnancy gives your mouth some extra love needs, so don't let those gums feel left out.
If you've been playing hide-and-seek with the dentist, it's time to throw in the towel and schedule that appointment. Let your pearly whites know you've got their back!

Ready for a second-trimester escape? Go you!
Vacations before the baby bump grows like a proud balloon are pure genius. Just make sure to run it by your doc first – they're your travel buddies on this adventure. If a plane's in the cards, peek at the airline's pregnancy policy to be the savvy flyer you were born to be.

Baby Steps to Birth
Hunt down a birthing school that vibes with your style and isn't a world away from your turf. Enroll in a course that's like a GPS for navigating the journey of childbirth.

Week 15 – 4th month– 2nd Trymester!
Your baby

Baby's Got Style: The 15-Week Fashion Show!
Guess what? You've hit the 15-week mark on this incredible pregnancy adventure, and your baby is now strutting around at the size of a grapefruit – talk about growing like a champ!

So, picture this: inside your cozy baby universe, a little sculptor is at work, molding those adorable facial features. The ears are taking their rightful place, settling in low on the sides of that precious head. It's like your baby's getting all dolled up for their grand entrance.

Oh, and speaking of style!
Your little one's hair plans are underway but here's the beauty of it – every baby's story is a bit different. Some arrive with a full-on head of hair, while others are as smooth as a jazz saxophone for those first few months.
But there's a common thread: the lanugo, or fetal moss. It's like a soft, downy layer of hair that's there to keep your baby cozy and comfy in its tiny world.

Secret veils
Now, let's talk about skin – it's like a delicate veil covering a fascinating secret. Those intricate blood vessels beneath the surface are on a mission, transporting a whopping 100 liters of blood every single day.
All thanks to your baby's heart that's growing and pumping like a superstar.

Get ready for a show – your little gymnast is hitting the mat!
Even though you might not be feeling it just yet, your baby's a budding acrobat, twirling and flipping in that amniotic sac. It's like having a backstage pass to the most adorable circus.

So there you have it, mama-to-be, your baby's got moves, style, and a heart that's pumping like a rock concert. Every week is a new chapter in this amazing story, and you're the author making it all come to life!

Your body

Ah, the wonderful world of the pregnancy belly – it's like a canvas telling your unique story. For most moms-to-be, this beautiful bump starts to peek out between the magical 13th and 16th weeks of this adventure. But hey, remember that every journey is its own masterpiece.

Now, if you're ready to shout your news from the rooftops, that emerging baby belly might just be the perfect spotlight. It's like a visual confirmation of the beautiful secret you're carrying. On the other hand, if you're holding onto your secret for a little longer, those loose-fitting shirts and cozy sweaters are your go-to accomplices in keeping things under wraps.

And speaking of news, guess what's making a grand exit? Chronic fatigue!
For many lucky moms-to-be, it's like waving goodbye to the never-ending yawns and welcoming a burst of energy that's ready to paint the town. If you're part of this energy-fueled club, embrace it like a warm sunbeam after a rainy day.

Now, it's time for action!
Exercise becomes your sidekick, prenatal classes your secret weapon, and local parenting clubs your new hangout. And let's not forget the baby's room – it's like a blank canvas waiting for your creative touch. Whether you're hitting the yoga mat, joining a support group, or picking out the perfect shade of paint, these are the chapters where you start turning your dreams into reality.

So there you go, mama-to-be! It's all about embracing the belly, riding the energy wave, and diving into this new chapter with enthusiasm. Your story's unfolding, and you're the one holding the pen.

Ah, the world of pregnancy changes – from that radiant glow to the unexpected twists!
Let's dive into a couple of chapters you might be encountering:

First up, we've got the puffiness party – aka, swollen feet and legs.
You're feeling like a water balloon parade, with your feet, ankles, and calves leading the way. Your hands and arms might even join in, though they're more like the VIP guests. Blame it on the water retention that's decided to set up shop in your body. But there's a hormone villain in this tale too – relaxin. This sneaky character loosens ligaments and gives bones a bit of a stretch, often leading to swollen feet. But don't worry, your feet are in good company – you're not alone in this puffiness journey.

The Never-Ending Nasal Party: A Pregnancy Tale of Hormones and Hydration
Blame those hormones – they're the mischievous masterminds behind the mucous membrane's grand congestion plan. But guess what? Staying hydrated is like your VIP ticket to this party. And if the congestion's really giving you a hard time, saline nasal drops are your trusty sidekick, swooping in for the rescue.

Pregnancy Amnesia: Scatterbrained Club
Ever feel like your mind's taken a vacation? Forgetting things left, and right? Blame it on the hormonal symphony, sleepless nights, and the stress that sometimes crashes the party. When it comes to whether pregnancy does a number on memory and brainpower, experts are split. But if you're in the "scatterbrained club," you're definitely not alone.

Here's a tip: Embrace the magic of tech! Those notepad and reminder functions on your tablet or smartphone can be your trusty companions in the quest to keep tasks in check. And if you're curious, dive into whether "momnesia" is a true tale or a myth. You've got the power to navigate distraction during pregnancy like a pro.

Uninvited and Grumpy: The Lower Back Pain Party Crashers of Pregnancy

Now, lower back pain – it's like the grumpy guest that shows up uninvited. But here's the good news: you're not alone in this party either. Many moms-to-be find themselves dealing with this unwelcome guest for around 15 weeks. Say hello to good posture and well-shaped shoes with low heels – they're like the bouncers keeping the pain at bay. And those back-strengthening exercises? They're your secret weapon against this villainous pain.

Gums Gone Wild: Pregnancy's Dramatic Dental Dilemma

Brushing and flossing might feel like a reenactment of a dramatic movie scene with a touch of bleeding. Thanks, pregnancy hormones! They've decided to throw a bit of inflammation and gum disease into the mix, often starring gingivitis. But don't stress – while the storyline might not be ideal, you've got the power to play the hero. Saltwater rinses and a soft-bristled toothbrush are like your trusty allies.

And here's a pro tip: Your friendly superhero dentist can give you personalized advice for your oral hygiene during this journey.
Your sparkling smile deserves the red carpet treatment!

Spider Veins: Pregnancy's Unwanted Stars

Pregnancy's got its own set of surprises, and here's one – the expansion of blood volume leading to the grand debut of "spider veins." These are those delicate, branching threads of red or blue that might decide to make a cameo on your legs or even your face. But don't worry, you've got a secret weapon – exercise and elevate those legs like you're giving them a VIP experience. This dynamic duo can improve blood flow and keep those spider veins at bay. And guess what? They often take a bow and exit the stage after childbirth.

UTIs in Pregnancy: A Bump in the Road

Pregnancy can make you a bit more susceptible to these pesky infections. If you find yourself experiencing pain or discomfort while peeing, an urgent need to empty your bladder, or even a fever or back pain, it's time to hit the speed dial with your pregnancy doctor. They're like the superheroes of your journey, ready to swoop in and save the day. Antibiotics might be on the prescription pad to prevent these infections from escalating into more serious issues, like bladder or kidney infections.

And the grand finale – weight gain.

Remember those mornings when nausea was your not-so-welcome companion? Well, say goodbye to that, because you've probably hit the appetite jackpot. Your baby's growing like a champion, and that belly of yours might be rounding out like a proud sculpture.

But hey, every curve tells a unique story.

Things to consider

Changing Desires and Hormones

Ah, the dance of desire! Your desires and your partner's might be doing the cha-cha in different directions, especially during pregnancy. Blame those hormones, the growing bump, and all the changes happening in your life. It's all part of the adventure, and it's okay! Just remember, open conversations are like the secret ingredient in this mix.

Choosing Where to Give Birth

Have you thought about where you want to welcome your baby? Experts give a big thumbs-up to hospitals and accredited birthing centers as safe choices. But here's the game-changer – get personalized insights from your doctor. Once you've made that decision, why not take a tour? It's like scoping out your own little piece of baby paradise before the big day. And guess what? The second trimester is your prime time for planning – from comfort strategies during labor to figuring out who'll be your partner in the birth adventure.

Intimacy and Communication

Let's talk about the big "S" word – sex during pregnancy. Here's the scoop – for most moms-to-be, it's a green light. But here's the catch: communication. It's like the golden key to the intimacy castle. Chat openly with your partner about your needs and feelings, and if any questions arise, don't hesitate to consult your doctor. They're like the wise mentors of your love story.

Gender Reveal on the Horizon

The suspense is building – the day to possibly discover your baby's gender during the mid-pregnancy ultrasound is just around the corner. It's like that exciting twist in your pregnancy story, happening somewhere between 18 to 22 weeks. Get ready to find out if you're having a mini superhero or a sweet little princess!

Musical Bonding Time

Guess who's tuning into the world? Your little one! With those ears picking up on sounds, it's like they're attending their own private concert. So why not have a daily music session? Imagine you and your baby relaxing and grooving to your favorite tunes. It's not just about music – it's a stress-busting strategy too.

The power of melodies is real, mama-to-be!

Staying Active and Energized

Keeping your energy levels up and your body in great shape during pregnancy is like preparing for a marathon. The secret? Moderate-intensity exercises, like walking, swimming, or yoga. But before you start channeling your inner athlete, it's superhero time – consult your doctor for the green light on any new workout plan. Walking is like the star of the show – easygoing, refreshing, and totally doable.

Bonus points if you team up with a friend or family member for some company. Oh, and for extra credit, consider using an app to track your daily activity. It's like having a personal fitness sidekick that counts your steps.

So there you have it, mama-to-be!

From bonding through music to navigating intimacy and anticipating the gender reveal, you're on a journey filled with surprises and shared moments.

Week 16 – 4th month– 2nd Trymester!
Your baby

Imagine your baby, all cozy in their apple-sized haven. At 16 weeks, they're about 11 centimeters from head to limb, and weighing in at around 113 grams. It's like a pocket-sized bundle of growth!

Brace yourself for a potential milestone – those first baby moves!
Between now and the 20th week, you might start feeling those tiny flutters. But hey, no pressure. Every pregnancy's got its own rhythm. And if those flutters feel a bit like a mystery, it's all part of the baby dance – they're like the gentlest of reminders that a tiny star's on the move.

Guess who's hitting the baby gym?
Your little one's muscles are gearing up for a strength show. The head's on the rise, arms and legs are coordinating their moves – it's like a baby ballet happening in there.

Hold up, ears!
Your baby's ears are on a journey to their final destination. And guess what? Your tiny maestro might just be catching some early tunes. Yep, your voice or those sweet lullabies could be making their way to those developing ears. So go ahead, serenade that belly!

Ready for some gender-guessing games?
Around this time, that "midterm" ultrasound could spill the beans on your baby's gender. If your baby's feeling shy and hiding their secret, don't worry. You might have to wait a bit longer to know whether it's Team Blue or Team Pink. It's like a suspenseful movie plot!

Your body

You're almost at the midpoint of your pregnancy journey – how awesome is that?

Hey there, Weight Watcher!

Wondering about those pregnancy pounds? If you kicked off your pregnancy with a healthy BMI (that's between 18.5 and 24.9), the scale's likely tipping at around a kilogram per week until the grand delivery. If you're feeling puzzled about the perfect pregnancy weight, don't hesitate to reach out to your doc. They're like your weight whisperer, and they've got the guidance you need.

And hey, a nutritionist can also be your secret weapon for cracking the healthy eating code during this special journey. It's like having your own personalized roadmap to stay on track!

Guess what? Your baby bump's gearing up for its grand entrance!

By the 16th week, it's like a VIP guest making their debut. While every mom's journey is one-of-a-kind, it's not uncommon for that belly to start making its presence known. And as it grows, why not treat yourself to some comfy maternity clothes?

Sleep, Sweet Sleep: Ready to cozy up for some quality Z's?

Sleeping might be a bit of a puzzle as your bump grows, but here's a tip: Side snoozing's the way to go. Belly sleeping might not be as comfy, and back snoozing can put extra pressure on that blood-returning vena cava. The left side's the hero here – it amps up circulation, sending that golden blood flow to your little one and your vital organs.

Pillows are your sleep sidekicks – tuck one between your knees and another to support your belly for added comfort. Can't seem to find the perfect position? Your doc's got your back – give 'em a call for some sleep-saving tips!

How you might feel in week 16?

Back Pain Dance

Oh, the familiar dance of lower back pain – it's like an unexpected guest at the party. But don't let it steal the spotlight! Warm baths and gentle stretches are your backstage passes to comfort. Keep an eye on your posture, slip into low-heeled shoes for the perfect dance partners, and hey, staying active with safe exercises can be your groove for beating back that backache.

Glow Getter: Ready to shine like a star?

Welcome to the world of "pregnancy glow"! Your skin's getting the VIP treatment with extra blood volume and those pregnancy hormones putting sebum production in overdrive.

Result? Your skin might be blushing and gleaming like a true superstar. While many moms embrace this radiant phase, a few uninvited guests might show up too.

Nosebleed Blues

Do you feel like your nose is staging a solo act? Don't worry, you're not alone! Those pesky nosebleeds might make an appearance around week 16, thanks to your upgraded circulation and hormone levels. While they're a normal part of the pregnancy package, they're definitely not the most fun.

- **Nose-nurturing Hacks:** Keep those nosebleeds in check by cranking
- up the humidity indoors – it's like a spa day for your nostrils. And hey, a touch of Vaseline on the edges of your nose can work wonders too. And when it comes to blowing your nose, take it easy and be gentle – it's like giving your nose a little TLC.

Whoa, is the world doing a twirl?

Dizziness might decide to make an appearance during this pregnancy party. Blame it on those hormones doing a dance with your circulation. But fear not, you're not alone in this dizzy ride!

- **Stay Hydrated:** Keep your cool by keeping those fluids flowing. Staying hydrated can be like a superhero power against dizziness.
- And if you're standing for a while, give yourself a break – prolonged standing isn't your dizziness's favorite jam.

- **Lying Low:** If the dizziness strikes, why not take a seat – or better yet, lay down on your side? It's like giving your body a breather to catch its balance.

And hey, if dizziness wants to join you during your exercise routine, don't hesitate to let your doctor know.
Safety first, right?

Things to consider

Tag Along Dark Spots

Say hello to melasma, those temporary dark spots that might pop up – they're like the rain on your glow parade. But don't worry, they often fade after your little one's big debut. And oh, the acne may decide to join the party too, making an occasional appearance. Not to fret – a gentle face wash twice a day can help you bid adieu to those party crashers.

Dental Diplomacy

If your pearly whites need a little extra TLC, schedule those dental treatments for this trimester. Haven't had a checkup in the last six months? Consider this your dental wake-up call. A healthy smile for you and your little one is a win-win.

Picture-Perfect Moments: Your baby bump is stealing the show!

Capture those moments with milestone cards for an adorable photo diary of your growing belly. Whether you share them on social media or keep them as cherished keepsakes, these cards are like a memory time capsule.

Doctor's Orders - Time for a little chat with your doc:

AFP Test Tango

Thinking about the AFP test? It's like a prenatal detective story for spotting certain birth defects. Chat with your doctor to see if it's on the pregnancy radar. This blood test is usually done between weeks 16 and 18, and it's like a spotlight on conditions like Down syndrome and spina bifida. Dive into the discussion about benefits and possible considerations.

Amniocentesis Inquiry

If it's on your mind, ask your doctor about this procedure. It's like getting the backstage pass to check your baby's health. Whether it's recommended for you depends on your unique pregnancy journey.

Week 17 – 5th month– 2nd Trymester!
Your baby

Size Check
Your baby's like a tiny pear in there, measuring around 13 cm with that dark-lipped length (CRL). It's like they're crafting their way into the world, growing and expanding with every passing day.

Heat Master
Here's a cool fact – your baby's getting their own heat generator! It's like they're installing a layer of brown adipose tissue, like a cozy winter coat, right under their skin. As the pregnancy journey unfolds, this fat layer gets thicker, becoming their ultimate source of warmth. It's like a natural heater, keeping its internal temperature just right – a job that your trusty uterus has been handling perfectly so far!

Vernix, the Protector
Imagine this – your baby's like a little explorer, equipped with a special shield. Their sebaceous glands are secreting a magical potion called vernix – it's like
a sticky, whitish superhero cape for their skin. This "cape" is their shield against the effects of months spent swimming in the amniotic fluid. It's like a waterproof layer, protecting their skin from dryness and helping them stay cozy while regulating their body temperature.

Baby's Moves
It's like your baby's got some secret moves up their sleeve, or rather, in your belly. If you're on round two of this adventure, you might recognize the sensation more easily – it's like a familiar melody playing in the background. But don't worry if you're not feeling the groove just yet – in the coming weeks, your little acrobat might surprise you with sensations resembling butterfly wings or gentle burbling.

Hold onto your socks, mama
Your baby's toenails are like the tiniest work of art, growing away quietly! By the end of this month, your fingernails might just be reaching all the way to your toes, like a symphony of growth.
Get ready for a possible post-birth trim, just in case those nails decide to be overachievers!

Feet on the Move

Have you noticed your feet joining the growing party? It's like they're trying on a new size. Weight gain and the magical water-retaining powers of pregnancy might be behind this transformation. Here's a trick – treat your feet to a soothing cool water soak. And when you can, elevate those legs like you're giving them a VIP seat. It's like giving your feet a little vacation from the swelling.

Growing Placenta

Imagine your baby's personal nutrient and oxygen supplier – that's the placenta! It's like a bustling factory, growing rapidly to make sure your little one gets everything they need to thrive. And it's not just about providing – the placenta's also got a waste-removal job. It's like the ultimate multitasker in your pregnancy tale.

Breast Changes

It's like your body's preparing for the grand milk production show! Your breasts might be growing faster than a sunflower. Thanks to increased blood flow, they're getting ready to be milk-making powerhouses. You might even spot those dark veins making an appearance – like nature's art show. And guess what? Cup sizes might change, too. It's like a shopping spree for bras. For the perfect fit, consider getting advice from a bra-fitter, just to make sure everything's snug and comfy.

How you might feel in week 17?

Oh boy, how should we start this one...

Lower Back Troubles

Let's talk about your back – it's like the support system on this amazing journey. But as your uterus takes center stage and your body adjusts, your posture might start doing its own dance. This shift can put extra pressure on your lower back, leading to those occasional twinges of discomfort. It's like a temporary hitch in the rhythm of pregnancy.

Leg Cramp Intruders

Say hello to leg cramps – those pesky nighttime visitors. They're like the unwelcome sidekicks that might disrupt your sleep. Nobody's quite sure why they show up, but here's your defense strategy. Before bedtime, stretch those calves like a champ. And if they still decide to crash the party, give them a little massage. Staying hydrated and staying active are like the VIP passes to keeping those cramps at bay. And remember, comfy shoes are your sidekicks in this quest for comfort.

Heartburn and Indigestion Drama

Morning nausea might be taking a bow, but guess who's stepping onto the stage? It's heartburn and indigestion, making their appearance. These are like the surprise guests who stick around. But here's the strategy: think small, frequent meals instead of big feasts. Skip the spicy acts and opt for foods that play nice with your tummy.

And here's a pro tip: Slow down while chewing, and don't take the lying down position right after a meal. It's like the script for comfort during mealtime.

The Weighty Matter

Here's the scoop – as your pregnancy plot unfolds, so does the weight gain. And that extra load can sometimes cause your lower back to speak up. But guess what? You've got the tools to tame the discomfort. Think exercises and gentle stretches – they're like your backstage passes to soothing those aches. And if you want some extra comfort, consider a warm hug from a heating pad on the sore spots.

Hemorrhoid Hassles

Let's address the elephant in the room – or rather, the veins in the rectum. Hemorrhoids are like the uninvited guests at the pregnancy party. Those veins down there are getting extra cozy due to increased pelvic blood flow. While they often arrive later in the pregnancy plot, you can take some steps now to keep them at bay.

Think fiber-rich diet, staying hydrated like a pro, and regular exercise. If they do make an appearance, warm baths and avoiding prolonged sitting might be your secret weapons. But if the situation turns intense – like severe pain or bleeding – your doctor's like the hero to call.

Skin Sensations

Your skin's like the canvas for this pregnancy masterpiece, and it's stretching to accommodate your growing belly and breasts. But here's the thing – that stretch might come with an itch. It's like your skin's telling its own story. Stay hydrated like a champ and treat yourself to a moisturizing lotion morning and night. While you can't fully dodge the appearance of stretch marks, you can definitely give your skin some comfort.

Things to consider

Mystery of the Gender

The excitement's building up – who's that little soul you're nurturing? Is it a boy or a girl? The curiosity's like an extra beat in your heart. But here's the scoop – it might still be a bit early for a definitive answer. However, a special moment is coming up – the midterm ultrasound, shining its spotlight between the 18th and 22nd week of your pregnancy. It's like the grand unveiling if you choose to know before the big day.
But like any good story, there's a twist. Your baby's position in the spotlight plays a role. Sometimes they're the ultimate cooperators, and sometimes they're the stars of unpredictability. So while the doctor's like the detective with the ultrasound wand, your baby's the wild card.

Finding the Perfect Pediatrician

It's like searching for a superhero for your little one – the pediatrician! Take some time to start the hunt. Ask fellow parents for their trusted recommendations or check out the lineup of doctors at your chosen clinic. It's like building a team for your baby's future.

Partner in Crime

Pregnancy can be like a whirlwind, shaking up even the strongest relationships. But guess what? Your partner's your co-pilot on this adventure. Share your feelings, and involve them in the milestones – tests, prenatal activities, and baby prep. It's like a partnership dance to avoid any bumps on the road.
And remember, if things get complex, your doctor's got your back – they're like the relationship counselor who can help you find the right support.

Week 18 – 5th month– 2nd Trymester!

Your baby

From Yam to Yam-Sized: Baby's Weight Gain Secrets Revealed!
At 18 weeks, it's like holding a yam-sized bundle of joy.
Picture this – about 14 centimeters from top-of-head to pelvis-lowest, and tipping the scale at around 200 grams.

Meconium: The Grand Black-Tie Affair of Diaper Changes!
In the culinary corner, the baby's digestive system is in full R&D mode.
It's been sipping on amniotic fluid, giving its stomach and intestines a test run. Think of it as the ultimate taste test, as this fluid mingles with leftovers – like dead cells and secretions – to cook up a special concoction.

Voilà, meconium is served!

Baby's Fingerprint Artistry: Tiny Picasso in the Womb!
This week, the baby is getting artsy – developing its very own fingerprint lines. Those tiny fat pads forming on its fingers and toes are gearing up to create unique swirls, like miniature masterpieces etched in skin.

Baby's Ears: The World's Smallest Boomboxes
Your baby is turning into a little audiophile too. Around week 18, those ears are stepping away from the head, ready to catch some sound waves. They're gearing up to be the world's tiniest boomboxes, registering the symphony of life.

Gallbladder, the Gourmet Chef of Digestion: Baby's Got Taste!
Speaking of digestion, your baby's gallbladder is clocking in for duty at week 18. It's like the gourmet chef behind the scenes, ensuring that bile is on the menu for optimal nutrient digestion.

Baby's Got Moves: The Secret Handshake Inside the Womb!"
If this is your pregnancy debut, get ready for a little surprise party in your belly – the baby's debut moves! It's like a secret handshake, a gentle tickling that's just for you.
As the tiny tenant gets more space to groove, those movements will start to feel more like acrobatics. Soon, you might even get little kicks and jabs – it's like the baby saying, "Hello, I'm here and I'm ready to rock this womb!"
But hey, not every mom's dance floor has the same beat. Some moms might feel these moves earlier, especially if they're old pros at pregnancy. Others might have a more chill baby, taking their time to perfect their dance moves. So, if you're not feeling the baby boogie at 18 weeks, don't sweat it.

Blood Pressure: The Vanishing Act – Where's My Script, Body?
Meanwhile, in your body's backstage, your circulatory system is getting a makeover. With more blood pumping and blood vessels throwing open their doors, blood pressure might play the disappearing act and leave you feeling a bit lightheaded.

Swollen Feet: The Cinderella Conundrum of Pregnancy!
If you've noticed Cinderella's slipper is feeling a bit snug, it's not a fairy tale. Blame it on the edema – water retention's pesky cousin – that might pop up like an uninvited guest around this time.

Relaxin: The Hormone with a Split Personality – Pelvis vs. Feet!
Blame it on those tricky pregnancy hormones – they've got their own grand plans for your feet. One of the masterminds, relaxin, is pulling double duty. On one hand, it's throwing a party for the pelvis, loosening things up to make way for the baby's grand entrance. On the other hand, it's playing sneaky games with your feet's ligaments, making them more flexible and roomier, almost like your feet are saying, "Expand and conquer!"
But fear not, weary traveler of swollen feet – relief is just a footbath away. Cool water to the rescue, and a little rest with those legs reaching for the stars (or at least your comfy sofa).

First up, we've got "The Dizzinator"
Your heart's taken up a part-time job pumping extra hard, and your expanding uterus is like, "Hey blood vessels, let's squeeze a bit." Cue the occasional fainting act, especially if you decide to stand up in a hurry. Oh, and watch out for the low blood sugar dive too – it might just pull a disappearing act on you.
Solution? Rest, lie down like a starfish, or snack on some fruit – your body's secret weapon against dizziness.

Next, we've got "The Gentle Mover"
Your baby's practicing its moves, but it's still a tiny tango dancer. So, expect more like a gentle mush than a karate kick.

Now, let's not forget "Leg Cramp Central"
Those calf cramps are like surprise guests showing up at night. Stretch those calves before hitting the sack, guzzle water, and maybe throw in a warm bath, hot shower, or a massage for good measure.

Then we have "Nasal Nuisance"
Your hormones are having a party, and your mucous membranes are like, "Let's swell up and have some bleeding fun!" But don't worry, it's a common gig.

Lastly, presenting "Backache Extravaganza"
Your belly's growing, your hormones are having a laugh, and your lower back is like, "Help, I need a break!" Some good and comfy shoes, body stretches, and maybe a heating pad might be your backstage crew for this one.

Things to consider

Plot twist
In those rare cases when the mid-term ultrasound uncovers a plot twist in the plot – like potential placental dramas – your doctor's the virtuoso who will guide you through the notes of understanding and action, who will lead you to the right composition of precautions and strategies, ensuring your symphony of pregnancy remains harmonious.

Unsolicited Advice: Navigating the Sea of 'Expertise' on Your Pregnancy Journey!

From your mother-in-law to the grocery store cashier, it's like they've all earned their doctorate in doling out guidance. Take it all with a grain of humor-infused wisdom. No need to give a dissertation defending your choices. A simple "Thanks, I'll keep that in mind" is your one-size-fits-all response. Remember, most are well-meaning companions in your journey, even if their serenades are a bit off-key.

Who knows, amidst the bullcrap, you might just find a golden nugget of advice.

The culinary journey of pregnancy

Ah, pregnancy – the time when every morsel you eat becomes a star in the cosmic drama of nourishing your little one. Enter omega-3 fatty acids, the nutritional superheroes of this tale. They're not just regular nutrients; they're the headliners, the main event, the ones with all the cool moves. They're like the dazzling soloists stealing the spotlight, especially when it comes to supporting your baby's nervous system development.

But hold on, they've got encore performances too – boosting your immune system and kicking those blues to the curb.

To invite these nutritional divas into your daily act, turn your attention to salmon and other fatty fish. They're like the lead actors who deliver an unforgettable performance. And let's not forget our unsung heroes – flaxseeds, broccoli, and walnuts. They're like reliable sidekicks, always there to keep your dietary story in perfect harmony.

Now, let's chat about the calorie ballet

Yes, you're hosting a tiny superstar in your belly, but this isn't an all-you-can-eat buffet. Think of it as sharing the stage with a duet partner in your daily calorie intake. During the second trimester, the script calls for about 300 extra calories per day – a delightful addition that keeps the nutritional storyline engaging. It's like adding a light, well-rehearsed scene to your regular 2000-calorie performance – a petite sandwich and a sip of skim milk, executed with finesse.

Week 19 – 5th month– 2nd Trymester!
Your baby

Mango Marvel

Your baby's size is catching up to a juicy mango! At 19 weeks, they measure about 18 centimeters and weigh between 180 to 230 grams. Check in with your doc during this time to get a closer look at your little one's growth as they measure the uterine fundus height.

Smooth Operator

A unique baby accessory is in the works! Your baby's skin is getting a layer of protection – a waxy coating known as fetal smear. It's a mix of sebum, those tiny lanugo hairs, and discarded skin cells. This combo helps shield your baby's skin from the amniotic fluid they're hanging out in. Most of it will vanish before the big arrival, but some early birds might be born with a bit of extra coating.

Dreamland Discoveries

Around this point, your little one is getting into the groove of sleep cycles. They're starting to snooze and wake up in a more predictable pattern. They might even catch some Z's in response to movements and sounds. It's like a preview of the sleepless nights ahead, but oh-so-adorable!

Gender Gossip

For baby girls, their reproductive system is on point with a developed vagina, uterus, and fallopian tubes. They've got ovaries that start with more than six million primary egg cells, and by birth, this number will whittle down to around one million.

If it's a little boy on the horizon, his journey to masculinity is underway. His testes have already developed and producing testosterone since the 10th week. The outside package is also coming together with ongoing developments.

Guess what? Your belly is putting on its own little magic show

It is growing and rounding up like a champ! You might even be able to balance a bowl of popcorn on there soon! But along with this awesome baby belly comes some pesky discomforts like swollen feet, dizziness, and back pain.

But don't worry, these are just little reminders that your baby is on the way to superstar status – kicking and wiggling inside you!

Energizer Bunny

Feeling like you've got a turbo boost of energy? That's your supercharged pregnancy mode kicking in! But remember, while you might want to tackle a hundred things on your to-do list, don't forget to take a breather and recharge. Maybe start planning the ultimate baby shower or ticking off those adorable outfits from your baby's shopping list – all while still taking it easy.

You've got this!

Snooze Strategies

Let's face it – getting a solid night's sleep can be a bit of a mission with your growing belly. Sleeping on your back might feel like you're doing a yoga pose, and waking up dizzy isn't exactly the dream scenario.

Try cuddling up on your side with a pillow between your knees and another one under your bump.

And if you wake up on your back, just roll back onto your side – no biggie!

How you might feel this week?

Feeling like you're in a dizzy dance?

Your body's hormones and increased blood volume might be the choreographers. Sometimes a bit of lightheadedness or faintness can join the party too. If you're feeling a little weak, just lie down, and make sure you're sipping on that water. Hydration is key to keeping your moves smooth.

Stretching Pains

Your uterus is like a master architect, making room for your growing baby. But sometimes, as it expands, ligaments stretch and can cause a twinge of pain in your lower abdomen. Ouch! It might feel like a little jab when you change positions or stand up quickly. A little rest will give you some relief. But if that pain comes with fever, chills, pain while peeing, bleeding, or it's just too intense, don't hesitate to reach out to your doc.

Back in Action

That growing belly is like a spotlight, and it's shining right on your back! Your expanding uterus and those sneaky hormones are teaming up to give you some back pain. As your center of gravity shifts, those back muscles are working overtime.
But fear not! You can combat this with stretches and strengthening exercises for your back muscles. If you're into fashion statements, try an abdominal support garment. And if you really want to up your game, an electric pillow might be your new BFF

Glow and Grow

Your hormones are like little artists, painting unique patterns on your skin! Brown spots on your nose, cheeks, and forehead might pop up – don't worry, it's just chloasma or the "mask of pregnancy." And that's not all – they're also giving you a special linea nigra, a black line running down your belly. Both of these art pieces will eventually fade post-baby, but be sure to avoid the sun or use sunscreen to keep them from getting too vivid.

Nosey Business

Feeling like your nose is throwing a tantrum? It might be rhinitis, a fancy term for a runny or stuffy nose. Blame it on those hormones again, plus the increased blood production. They're causing your nasal mucous membranes to swell up, leading to rhinorrhea (fancy word for a runny nose) and even nosebleeds. Stock up on tissues and maybe a humidifier to soothe those irritated passages.

Midterm Ultrasound

Around 19 weeks, a midterm birth ultrasound can provide significant information about your baby's development. It's a non-invasive way to assess their growth, anatomy, and overall well-being.

Time to get your groove on, mama-to-be!

Staying active during your pregnancy can be like giving your body a little love tap. Think about it – regular, moderate exercise can be like a sunshine boost for your well-being and the whole pregnancy journey. Whether you're rocking walks, doing some mermaid-style swimming, striking yoga poses, or channeling your inner Pilates pro, these activities are like a customized playlist for pregnant ladies. Just remember to give your doc a high-five before you hit the dance floor – especially if you're new to these moves.

Let's give those back muscles some extra TLC

As your body's creating this baby masterpiece, your back muscles might feel like they're doing the Cha-Cha with some strain. But fear not! Bust out some exercises that target those back muscles, and you'll have your very own backup dancers helping to ease any discomfort. Your doctor's like the dance instructor in this routine, showing you the moves that'll hit the spot without missing a beat.

Let's talk about stress

Exercise is like the ultimate stress-buster playlist. It's like hitting the "chill" button while grooving to the pregnancy beat. Plus, joining a squad of fellow expectant parents in a support group is like having a backstage pass to swapping stories and tips on the pregnancy tour. It's like finding your own fan club full of comrades who totally get it.

VIP Pass

Imagine joining a club where everyone's got that same VIP pregnancy pass – that's support groups in a nutshell! Whether you're high-fiving fellow parents in person or swapping stories online, it's like finding your crew for this crazy journey. They're like the extra tracks on your pregnancy playlist – you learn from each other, share laughs, and build that "we're in this together" vibe.

Oooohhhh, we're halfway there (Good ol' Bon Jovi knew what he was signing about)!
Congratulations, you're now at the midway mark of your pregnancy, and there's a lot to cheer about!

Check out these highlights below for some exciting news:

From Mini to Jumbo!
Your 20-week superstar is about as big as a jumbo bell pepper. Their crown-rump length is around 15 centimeters, and their weight ranges from 255 to 312 grams – which means they'd still fit comfortably in your palms.

Baby's Got a Cute Nose! Just Wait Till You See the Rest
Your 20-week-old baby is shaping up to be a real cutie – facial features, including that adorable nose, are starting to take form.

Thumb Wrestling in the Womb
Your baby's sucking reflex is revving up, and you might catch them giving their tiny thumb a taste test.

Lights, Camera, Snooze!
Their sleep-wake rhythm is becoming more consistent. And guess what? Outside noises might even be enough to wake up this little snoozer.

It's not just about looks
Their skin is leveling up, with added layers and a protective waxy coating called fetal smear. It's like their own personal shield against the amniotic world.

Meet Meconium
That's the fancy term for the greenish-black, sticky substance their digestive system is busy producing. It's going to hang out in their intestines until showtime.

The brain power is real

Your baby's brain development is in turbo mode, especially in the zones responsible for their senses.

Ah, the grand unveiling of the baby's visage!

At the wondrous 20-week ultrasound, you might find yourself face-to-face with your little one's actual face for the very first time. Those early genetic ultrasounds were like the sneak peek trailers, but now, it's the main event – a true cinematic moment of parenthood.

Remember, this is your chance to request a VIP pass to the ultrasound photo gallery. Yes, that's right – ask for a printout of your baby's first-ever photo shoot.

Think of it as the inaugural snapshot for your baby's future album. You're starting the collection with the first chapter – the prenatal phase. As the chapters unfold, you'll have a visual narrative of your baby's journey from the womb to the world.

And just imagine, in a few moons, you'll have a sequel to add – the post-birth extravaganza.

Your body

Feeling the flutter

Around the 20-week mark of your pregnancy, you might start sensing the first delicate movements of your little one down in your belly. These sensations are often described as a gentle flutter or bubbling.

But don't fret if you haven't felt them just yet – it's perfectly normal! The timing of these first encounters with your baby and the way you perceive them can vary widely among different women.

After all, each pregnancy is as unique as a snowflake.

Hiccups in the Womb

As the weeks go by, you're in for quite the show. Alongside the spinning, somersaulting, and kicking, you might also experience rhythmic twitches – those are the unmistakable hiccups of your tiny bundle! Many babies get hiccups while still in the womb, likely due to their developing diaphragm getting into practice mode.

Just remember, there's no need to worry – it's all part of the adorable, harmless journey of your baby's growth.

Measuring Up: The Uterine Fundus Height Test Explained

As you approach week 20, you might be curious about the prenatal tests that lie ahead. During your regular check-ups, your doctor may start performing a special measurement called the uterine fundus height test. This involves measuring the distance from your pubic bone to the top of your uterus.

This measurement serves as a helpful indicator of the pregnancy's progress.

By the twentieth week, the top of your uterus should be aligned with your umbilicus (belly button), and the measurement from the bottom of your uterus should typically fall between 18 and 22 centimeters.

Here's a fascinating tidbit:

The measurement from the bottom of your uterus, expressed in centimeters, actually matches the number of weeks you've been pregnant. So, at 20 weeks, this measurement should be around 20 centimeters. It's a neat way to track your pregnancy's growth!

Double Trouble: Twin Pregnancy Belly Expansion Mode

If you happen to be expecting twins, brace yourself for a more rapid belly expansion compared to a single pregnancy. Twins tend to keep things exciting and dynamic!

What symptoms can you expect in week 20?

Ah, welcome to the delightful world of the 20th week of pregnancy symptoms!

Pregnancy Brain Fog's Grand Entrance

Ever feel like your brain's on a little vacation while you're trying to focus? Blame it on the pregnancy brain fog. But fear not, the superhero solution is creating mission-critical checklists and reminder notes. Stick 'em on your fridge, or your mirror, or just set up a digital army of reminders on your trusty phone.

Lower Back Pain: Carrying Joy and a Baby Bump

Your growing baby belly is like a backpack full of joy, and your back is feeling the weight, especially after a day's adventure. Rock some comfy, well-shaped shoes with a hint of heel, stretch those back muscles like a pro yogi, and if you're feeling fancy, consider a pregnancy brace to give your back some extra TLC.

Constipation: When Pregnancy and Slow Digestion Collide
Ah, the joys of pregnancy hormones and that growing bundle of joy in
your belly teaming up to slow down your digestive system. But fear not,
hydration and a fiber-rich diet can be your constipation-busting
superheroes

Congested Nose and Nosebleeds: Hormones' Party in Your Nasal Passages
Your hormones are in overdrive, and your nasal mucous membranes are
partying like it's the season of swelling and drying out. Enter the
congested nose and occasional nosebleeds. Combat this with a
humidifier's magical mist and the all-powerful hydration game.

Swollen Feet: The Relaxin-Induced Balloon Feet Party
Let's talk about the Cinderella moments when your feet decide they want
to party and puff up like balloons. You can thank the hormone relaxin for
this enchanting feat. It's the hormone that gets your joints in the party
mood for labor, but your feet also get an invite to this ballooning
extravaganza.

Try giving your feet the royal treatment by elevating them on a plush
cushion throne, and if they're still having a blast in the swelling party,
treat them to shoes a size larger for maximum comfort.

Next steps

Ah, it's time for the grand cinematic event of your pregnancy - the **Midline
Ultrasound Extravaganza!**

Grab your popcorn and let's dive in:

- **Lights, Camera, Ultrasound:** Between weeks 18 and 22, you'll be the
  star of your own ultrasound show. This high-tech performance is like
  a blockbuster for your baby's development. The doctor takes center
  stage, measuring the baby's size, and position, and giving a thumbs-up
  to those growing bones and organs.

- **Action-Packed Details:** Get ready for some behind-the-scenes action! This ultrasound doesn't hold back - it estimates your baby's age, weight, and even checks out their fancy moves and heart rate. Plus, it's all about the backdrop – your placenta's position and the amount of amniotic fluid in the studio.

- **Gender Reveal:** Hold onto your seats! This is the moment when your baby's gender takes the spotlight. The doctor might just let the cat out of the bag... or should we say, the baby out of the belly! But if you're all about suspense, give them a heads-up if you want the surprise to stay under wraps.

- **Burning Questions:** Feeling like a curious movie critic? Don't hesitate to ask your pregnancy doctor for the director's cut. They're your go-to for all things ultrasound-related, ensuring you're in the loop and ready for the next scene.

- **The Sweet Spot:** Welcome to the trimester sweet spot, where the morning sickness is on hiatus and the baby belly hasn't turned you into a walking obstacle course just yet. It's the golden time for jet-setting.

- **Flexible Flow:** Roll out the red carpet for spontaneity. Ditch the strict itinerary and embrace the "go with the flow" vibe. Your mood might change faster than a Hollywood plot twist, and that's totally okay.

- **Sky High or Road Trip:** Ready for takeoff? If you're planning to hop on a plane, get the green light from your doc and learn the airline rules (they're like the script, everyone's got their version). Remember, stretching your legs and staying hydrated are your new on-set priorities.

- **Globe-Trotter Tips:** Whether you're on a bus, train, car, or soaring through the skies, make pit stops for leg stretching. Snack like it's your job, and carry your medical records like a VIP pass – just in case.

- **Pre-Adventure Prep:** Before your grand exit, hit up your pregnancy doctor for a pre-adventure checkup. It's like your final script review, making sure you're set for a blockbuster journey.

Next up is a **Baby Gear Labirynth!**
Navigating the world of baby gear is like entering a labyrinth of choices –
cribs, strollers, car seats, oh my!
But fear not, for the wise wanderer knows the secrets to choose the best
for their mini-adventurer.

Here's your map to mastering the art of baby gear shopping:

- **Quest for Reviews:** Just as a knight consults ancient scrolls before
  embarking on a quest, read product reviews. The tales of other parents
  hold wisdom and warnings that can guide your choices.

- **Seek the Council:** Call upon the council of fellow parents, the wise
  sages who've been through the trenches of baby gear warfare. Their
  tales of victory and defeat will steer you clear of pitfalls.

- **The Crib Conundrum:** When choosing a crib, consider it the castle
  where your tiny royal shall slumber. Sturdy build and safety reign
  supreme in this kingdom of sleep.

- **Stroller Quest:** The stroller, your trusty steed, must be swift and
  versatile. Maneuverability and storage space will make your travels
  with your baby
  a breeze.

- **Car Seat Wisdom:** For safe travels, invest in a car seat that's worthy of
  guarding your little explorer. Check for safety ratings and make sure
  it's a snug fit for your carriage. With reviews as your compass and
  fellow parents as your guides, you'll navigate the realm of baby gear
  with confidence.

Your quest for the perfect crib, stroller, and car seat shall be a tale of
triumphant choice-making!

Week 21 – 6th month– 2nd Trymester!
Your baby

Ahoy, captain!
It's the 21st-week voyage of pregnancy, and your little sailor's growing like a banana on steroids! Yep, you heard right. Picture a banana-sized baby, measuring about 22 centimeters, and weighing between 283 and 368 grams. That's one hearty banana, I tell you!

Baby's Heartbeat: The Mini Dance Party Inside
Your baby's got a beat that's loud enough for a stethoscope to catch, but spotting it amidst your own heart's rhythm might need some detective skills. Listen for the faster tempo – we're talking 120-160 beats per minute, a heartbeat that's practically keeping up with galloping horses. Giddy up!

Guts and Glory: Baby's Digestive System Gearing Up
The baby's digestive system is gearing up for its debut. Swallowing small sips of amniotic fluid? Check. And those blood cells? They're making a shift from the liver and spleen production line to the bone marrow department. It's like your little one's getting ready for a career change even before they clock in for their first day on Earth!

Sleep Expert in the Making: Your Baby's Preferred Snooze Position
Ultrasound studies reveal they might even have their preferred snoozing position already – it's like they're setting up camp for the comfiest sleep in there.

Tiny Fingers and Toes: Fully Formed and Ready to Wave
But hold on, the star of the show is those teeny fingers and toes. They're fully formed and ready for some waving and wiggling. And guess what? Those fingers have fingerprints! Yep, even before they've rocked up to the outside world, they're already leaving their mark.

Thumbs-Up for Thumb-Sucking: Your Baby's Favorite Pastime
Oh, and did I mention your baby's turning into a thumb-sucking aficionado? It's their current favorite pastime, and if you're lucky enough to have an ultrasound scheduled, you might catch them in action.

Turning Up the Heat, One Hot Flash at a Time
Oh, the joys of pregnancy! As if heartburn and indigestion haven't been your sidekicks since the first trimester, now the growing uterus is like, "Hey, let's turn up the heat!" Yep, that's right, the expanding baby abode is pressing on your stomach, throwing a curveball at your digestive harmony.
Who knew pregnancy could turn you into your very own human oven? But wait, there's more!

Extra Pounds and Their Friends: Aches and Discomforts
Extra pounds are joining the party, and they're bringing their friends – aches, and discomforts that seem to pop up in all sorts of unexpected places.

But hey, don't let these surprises rain on your pregnancy parade! After all, a little discomfort is just a footnote in the grand adventure of growing a tiny human!

Possible symptoms in week 21

Ah, the magical 21st week of pregnancy, where discomforts seem to be auditioning for a leading role in your daily life.

Back pain: The Uninvited Guest of Pregnancy's 21st Week
Back pain, my dear friend, has RSVP'd for the party, settling in the lumbosacral region. And guess what? Your expanding belly has got the whole center of gravity thing going on, causing your lower spine to do a little forward shimmy.
It's like a recurring character in this grand production, but fear not, there are some backstage tricks to ease its presence. When you take a seat, consider giving your feet a little elevation with a footrest. And if you find yourself standing in the spotlight for a while, let one foot take a break on a small stool to give your lower back a breather. And when the curtain falls on the day, a warm bath might be your standing ovation for relief.
If the pain lingers like an encore, don't hesitate to call your doctor for some expert advice.

Heartburn: The Acidic Surprise Party in Your Esophagus

Heartburn makes its entrance with a grand flourish. Your superstar uterus is putting pressure on your stomach, while those sneaky pregnancy hormones decided to casually loosen the valve between your esophagus and stomach. Result? Acidic surprise party in your esophagus and everyone's invited!

Relaxin: The Hormone Behind Cinderella's Slipper Game

Meet relaxin – the hormone that's all about giving your joints and ligaments a relaxation vacation so your pelvis can get ready for the grand labor finale. But guess what? It might also be the culprit behind your feet playing Cinderella's slipper game, growing mysteriously larger.

Leg Cramps: The Encore You Didn't Ask For in the Second Trimester

Yes, those calf calves might decide to serenade you with a crampy symphony, especially when the curtain falls on the second trimester. Nighttime seems to be their favorite stage, so stretching before the bedtime bow, keeping hydrated like a pro, or even indulging in a warm bath or shower can be your secret weapon against these unexpected leg-cramp encore performances.

It's all part of the show, my dear!

Stretch Marks: Nature's Reminders of Your Skin's Elastic Odyssey

As your belly transforms into a canvas of life, you might notice the artistic arrival of stretch marks – those reddish, brownish, pinkish, or purplish streaks that have decided to make an appearance.

Picture them as nature's little reminder that your skin is making its best impression of a rubber band during this grand performance. They might pop up on your abdomen, hips, thighs, buttocks, and even the prized real estate of your breasts.

Fear not, for the diligent application of moisturizing lotion can be your knight in shining armor, providing relief to your skin that's stretching like a yoga master, and soothing those itchy sensations.

Hot Flashes: Pregnancy's Fiery Hormonal Circus

Let's welcome the sensation of hot flashes. Thanks to those hormones (they just can't seem to resist a good performance), and a metabolism that's decided to kick things up a notch, you might be feeling like a one-woman furnace. Don't worry – in the midst of this hormonal circus, remember to keep cool with loose clothing, stay hydrated, and maybe even strike a fan-assisted diva pose for added flair.

Vitamin B: The Superhero Supporting Your Pregnancy Plot
Now, let's talk about the vitamins making cameo appearances in your pregnancy plot. Vitamin B, the energy booster of the nutrient world, is here to support your little star's development, give a nod to vision, and even give a thumbs up to the placenta and other tissues. Your pregnancy supplement might be a trusty sidekick in the B vitamin realm, but you can also summon them from sources like liver, pork, poultry, bananas, and beans.

Choline: The Unsung Hero of Your Pregnancy Nutrient Crew
And speaking of nutrients, let's give a round of applause for choline – a nutrient that's joining the backstage crew. It might not be the headliner, but it's essential for both you and your growing star. While your body does a bit of choline production, it's like a magician's assistant – you need a bit more of its magic during pregnancy.
Keep an eye out for choline-rich performers like chicken, beef, eggs, milk, and peanuts in your dietary cast. They're here to ensure your baby's show goes on without a hitch!

Preparing for the Grand Debut: Setting the Stage for Your Little Star's Arrival
The upcoming weeks are like the dress rehearsal before the big show, so why not start prepping for the grand debut? Roll up your sleeves and take center stage in setting up the baby's room – it's like designing the backdrop for their first act. Craft a list of must-haves, set your budget as if you're planning a blockbuster, and assemble a wardrobe worthy of a star-studded layette.

Healthy Movement: Keeping Your Body in Harmony for the Grand Finale
Remember that movement is the key to a healthy performance. Your body is your instrument, and regular physical activity keeps the harmony alive. Consult with your director – ahem, doctor – to ensure you're choreographing safe exercises. From the rhythmic strides of walking to the serene flow of prenatal yoga, or even the elegant strokes of swimming, there's a whole repertoire of moves that'll keep you in perfect tune for the grand finale!

Week 22 – 6th month– 2nd Trymester!
Your baby

Buckle up for a brainy update!
Your baby's noggin is on a developmental rollercoaster, and it's like a symphony of nerve fibers taking the stage. These nerve endings are like the baby's hotline to the world, helping them sense their environment.

Get ready for some baby theatrics!
At 22 weeks, your little star might just put on a show. Imagine seeing those tiny arms and legs react to noise – it's like your very own sneak peek into their world of movement and sensation.

Baby's Sensory Makeover: Exploring the World One Touch at a Time
Your baby's sense of touch is getting a makeover too. It's like a sensory exploration adventure! They're all about experimenting – stroking their own body and maybe even giving that adorable thumb a good ol' suck. These little experiments are like their way of connecting with the world around them, one touch at a time.

Heat Team: Your baby's got a fat update for you
Right now, it's just around 1%. But don't worry, more layers of brown adipose tissue are on the way. Their mission? Generating and holding onto body heat. It's like your baby's personal heat squad getting ready for action!

Papaya Partner
Imagine a papaya – that's the ballpark size your baby's rocking at 22 weeks! Measuring in at about 19 centimeters, your little one's parietal and sitting length are making quite the statement. And let's talk weight – your baby's tipping the scale at around 450 grams.

Blink and Wink
Eyes might be shut, but they're not napping. Your baby's eyeballs are on the move, doing a little dance inside those closed lids. And guess what? Tear ducts are in the works and those baby brows? They're already showing some action, furrowing like a pro.
Bonus: Baby brows are sporting a white hue, with no pigment in sight.

Handy Dandy: Arm and leg alert!

Those little limbs are growing in proportion and your baby's making the most adorable moves. Think digging, grabbing, bending, and even some baby-style squeezing. The fingertip scene? It's got a new look, with tiny nails now fully covering those little fingers. They're like miniature works of art, but watch out – you might need some nail trimming duty post-birth to avoid accidental scratches.

Your body

Round and proud!

At 22 weeks, your belly's stepping into the spotlight – it's like the star of the show now. You might notice more and more folks giving you that knowing smile as they spot your baby bump. It's like a public debut, and the reactions of those around you are adding an extra layer of realness to this new chapter of life.

Let's talk about those curves, shall we?

Your body's putting on a pregnancy performance, and with those extra pounds and shifts in shape, it's totally normal to have some mixed feelings. Some days, you might be all about those pregnancy curves, and other days, you might feel like you're in uncharted territory. It's okay, these emotional ebbs and flows are as natural as the tides. If you're struggling, reach out – whether it's to a confidant close to your heart or your trusted doctor.

And don't forget, a combo of healthy eating and regular exercise can be like your superhero cape for feeling better.

Let's talk about that weight journey!

Remember, every mom's path is unique. If you're curious about the numbers on the scale at 22 weeks, it's all good to ask your doctor for some insight. They're like your pregnancy GPS, guiding you toward a healthy route.

If things seem a bit off track, your doctor can help map out some adjustments to steer you back in the right direction.

What's new in the symptoms world?

Pulse Power-Up

Your heart's got a workout routine too! During pregnancy, it's like your heart's hitting the gym, pumping 30-50% more blood than usual. Why? It's all about giving that placenta the green light to deliver extra oxygen and nutrients to your baby. So, if you find your heart racing a bit, don't worry – it's part of the pregnancy symphony. But if that pulse is racing to the point where you're short of breath or feeling uneasy, it's time to give your doc a call.

Pelvic Playground

Pregnancy's like a flexibility class for your joints, thanks to those hormones. But sometimes, all that stretching can lead to pelvic pain. The motto here is: take it easy. Avoid heavy lifting and don't stand for too long. Give those sore areas some TLC by avoiding extra strain.

Battle of the Burn

Ugh, heartburn – the uninvited guest that brings the burn to your chest and throat. Blame it on stomach acids having a wild party in your esophagus. And guess what? Pregnancy hormones are like the bouncers who relax the esophagus's muscles, letting those stomach acids crash the party.
But don't worry, you've got this. Opt for mini-meals throughout the day, stay upright after eating, and wave goodbye to spicy and fried foods.
If heartburn's playing the ultimate game of tag, it's time to call in the doctor squad.

Cramps and Contractions

Lower abdominal twinges and those "premonitory" contractions – also known as Braxton-Hicks contractions – are all part of the natural rhythm of pregnancy at 22 weeks. Your body's gearing up for the big day.
And that growing belly? It's like a stretching marathon for your muscles and ligaments. While these sensations are part of the journey, if things get seriously uncomfortable or confusing, it's a green light to reach out to your pregnancy doctor.
Better safe than sorry!

Hot Flash Frenzy

Feeling like a human radiator? You can thank those hormones and your turbo-charged metabolism for those hot flashes. But fear not, there's a cool-down strategy in play. Rock loose, comfy clothes, keep that hydration game strong with water and bring in the fan squad or air conditioner posse when things heat up. It's like having your own personal cooling system!

What's new in the symptoms world?

Birth Experience Boost

With the due date edging closer, it's like the spotlight's on preparing for the grand debut. Time to put on your research hat and explore the birthing options your hospital offers. Sit down with your doc, and ask about the magical world of pain relief methods – from anesthesia to massage to hydrotherapy. Want to create a birth plan? Pen down your preferences and dislikes. It's like crafting your own magical birthing recipe.

Birthing Squad

Who's your VIP guest at the birth bash? Think partner, family member, or BFF. And hey, ever heard of a doula? They're like birth superstars with special training to make your journey smoother. If you're thinking doula, start your search for references. Your doc or birthing school guru might have some leads. Then, set up face-to-face meetings – it's like the interview for your dream birthing team.

Breastfeeding Bliss

Eyeing the breastfeeding journey? Reach out for guidance – your doc's a great resource. And don't forget, fellow moms can drop some golden nuggets too. Ask around for clinic or lactation consultant suggestions. It's like building your breastfeeding support squad!

Intimate Insights

Let's talk about a topic that's often whispered about – sex during pregnancy. Good news: if you're in good health and your baby's development is on track, it's generally safe to continue your intimate adventures.

The key? Both of you feeling up for it and shaking off those worries about "baby damage."

Don't stress – your little one's like a VIP guest with protection from the amniotic sac and uterine muscles.

Desire's Diverse Dance

Your libido might just decide to take the spotlight and dance a little differently during this pregnancy gig.

Here's the scoop: Many moms-to-be find their desire peaking in the second trimester. It's like your energy levels rise and the first-trimester blues take a bow. But remember, every pregnancy's a unique ride, and your desire might take its own twist.

Spotlight on Safety

A bit of spotting or mild cramps after sex? It's like a gentle reminder that your body's in pregnancy mode. But if things start getting heavy in the bleeding or cramping department, it's your cue to reach out to your doctor.

And if your pregnancy's been sprinkled with complications – like the potential for preterm labor – your doctor might recommend pressing pause on the bedroom adventures.

Remember, it's all about comfort, communication, and doing what feels right for you and your partner. And yes, those intimate connections can absolutely coexist with your pregnancy journey.

Ah, week 23 – the curtain has risen on the sixth month of your grand pregnancy production, and you're cruising into the second trimester like a seasoned performer. It's almost time to flip the calendar page to the third act, but don't fret – you've got this!

Baby's Eggplant-Sized Charm

In the realm of numbers, your baby's weight is delicately balanced between 455 and 500 grams. As for measurements, their parietal and sitting length extend to a charming 20 centimeters.
While the size of each expectant mother's belly is as unique as her journey, the dimensions of your growing bundle of joy at 23 weeks paint a clearer picture. Imagine an adorable eggplant – that's about the size of your little wonder right now.

Music to Their Ears

In this exciting installment, your little one's sense of hearing takes center stage. Can you believe it? Those tiny ears are tuned in, and your voice is the star of the show. Reading stories, singing melodies, or simply sharing heartfelt whispers – it's all music to their ears. And don't forget to cue your partner in – their voice is a part of this serenade too, setting the stage for a symphony of family love.

The Real Show Behind the Scenes!

Behind the scenes, your baby's sleep is quite the spectacle. Napping away, they spend a whopping 80 percent of their rest time in a phase known as REM – the rapid eye movement phase. It's like a dreamland full of fluttering eyes and buzzing brain activity, setting the stage for growth and development.

The Unsung Hero of Pregnancy

Now, let's talk about that incredible amniotic fluid. It's like the unsung hero of this pregnancy play, creating the perfect ambiance for your baby's journey. Think of it as a protective buffer, maintaining a cozy temperature and cushioning their every move.

Baby's Got Moves

At 23 weeks of pregnancy, your baby's movements are likely becoming more noticeable to you, although the timing can vary for different expectant mothers. In the coming months, your healthcare provider might recommend that you keep track of your baby's movements by creating a diary and practicing "kick counting" at specific times.

To effectively monitor these movements, choose a consistent time when your baby is typically most active. Jot down each instance of movement you feel and record the time it takes for your baby to complete 10 movements.

If it takes more than 2 hours to perceive these 10 movements or if you observe any changes in your baby's usual patterns, don't hesitate to reach out to your doctor for guidance.

Your baby's activity level can offer valuable insights into their well-being.

Your body

Pregnancy is like a special edition of the "**Gaining Weight Game**," where the rules are different and the prize is a cute little bundle of joy!

On this journey, your weight gain is the scorecard, and the target range is usually around 4.5 to 7 kilograms. But don't worry, there's no losing here – just healthy gains.

Think of your doctor as the referee in this game. If your weight gain is speeding down the track faster than a race car, they might suggest tapping the brakes a bit. On the other hand, if you're taking a leisurely stroll through the weight gain park, they could give you the green light to enjoy a few more snacks.

Staying within the recommended weight gain range isn't just about fitting into those maternity jeans – it's about setting yourself up for a smoother ride during pregnancy and even post-delivery.

So, let your doctor be your coach, guiding you to the finish line with a healthy, happy baby in your arms.

And remember, you're playing for the ultimate prize!

How you might feel this week?

Your body's throwing you a pregnancy party complete with its own set of quirky symptoms!

Pain and Discomfort

Your belly's growing faster than the eyes of a kid in a candy store, which means muscle pain and the occasional headache might RSVP to the party. Want to soothe those aches? How about a warm bath or a gentle massage? But wait, before you raid your medicine cabinet for those trusty painkillers, make sure to check with your doc – your usual go-tos might need a pregnancy permission slip.

Oh, leg cramps, the uninvited guests of pregnancy

They might decide to drop by during the second and third trimesters but don't worry, you're not alone in this. You can counter their entrance by massaging your calves, doing some toe wiggles, or throwing in some calf stretches before bed. It's like giving your legs a little pre-sleep dance party. Remember, your pregnancy playlist is unique, and your symptoms are the dance moves that come with it.

If anything seems extra funky or if you're worried about those twirls, it's always smart to give your healthcare provider a shout-out for a personalized choreography check.

Things to consider this week

Essential guidelines to adhere to during pregnancy for both your safety and your baby's well-being. Let's break it down a bit further:

Limit Sodium Intake

Hey, I get it, pregnancy cravings can make you want to eat a whole bag of chips in one sitting. But here's the deal: too much salt can lead to bloating and high blood pressure. So, put down that salt shaker and opt for herbs and spices to jazz up your meals

Hygiene and Food Safety

Your superhero pregnancy hormones might make you feel invincible, but they don't protect you from foodborne illnesses. Wash your hands like you're performing surgery, cook your meats like you're auditioning for MasterChef, and steer clear of any dairy products that think "pasteurized" is optional.

Recognizing Food Poisoning

Food poisoning is the last party you want crashing your pregnancy parade. If you suddenly find yourself worshipping the porcelain throne with symptoms like fever, chills, and a stomach that's doing its own version of Riverdance, call your healthcare provider. They'll be your emergency hotline to save the day.

Stay Hydrated

Pregnancy is basically like growing a human rainforest, so hydration is key. Keep chugging that water like it's your job. And if you're getting tired of plain ol' H2O, throw in some lemon wedges or cucumber slices for some maternity mixology.

Variety of Nutrients

Variety is the spice of life, especially during pregnancy. Load up on colorful veggies, lean proteins, and whole grains. Think of your plate as a Picasso painting – the more colors, the better. Remember, these are not just pregnancy commandments – they're your ticket to a smooth and healthy journey through pregnancy.

But as always, your doc or a nutrition guru can help personalize this roadmap based on your unique pregnancy adventure. By following these food safety guidelines, you can significantly reduce the risk of foodborne illnesses and other potential health issues during your pregnancy journey. If you have any concerns or questions about specific foods, preparation methods, or dietary choices, don't hesitate to consult with your healthcare provider or a registered dietitian.

Watch out for another delightful aspect of pregnancy – high blood pressure!

Because who doesn't love the thrill of having your blood pressure constantly monitored by a doctor? It's like a never-ending rollercoaster ride, but instead of loops and drops, you get to worry about potential pre-eclampsia.

And let's not forget the glamorous symptoms of pre-eclampsia: edema (swelling that makes you feel oh-so-chic), and the pièce de résistance – protein in your urine. Why settle for a regular pregnancy when you can have protein-enhanced urine?!

Oh, and don't you worry – pre-eclampsia symptoms can hit the runway as early as 20 weeks into your pregnancy. Early detection, darling, is the name of the game. Get ready to flaunt your new accessories: spots in front of your eyes, the latest headache sensation, and the ever-fashionable sudden swelling of your hands and feet.

But wait, there's more!
If you're unlucky enough to experience nausea, sudden weight gain, or breathing problems call your doctor immediately, because untreated pre-eclampsia is the ultimate effing danger. It can mess with your placenta's VIP blood flow, and let's not forget the potential to become the next big thing in kidney, liver, brain, and eye damage.

So there you have it, folks – the not-so-glamorous world of pre-eclampsia. It's like a designer label for pregnancy complications. Remember, if you're spotting any of these haute symptoms, make that emergency call to your doctor.

Now, let's talk real talk – complications are like unicorns -rare (I am a believer!), but hey, better safe than sorry. Know what to look out for, just in case your pregnancy journey takes an unexpected turn. It's all about being prepared, like a pregnancy scout on a mission.

Happy thoughts!
Quick, before the sleep deprivation kicks in and you're running on caffeine and baby cries, let's squeeze in a pregnancy photo session. Hire a professional photographer or recruit a friend who somehow managed to nail Instagram aesthetics. I mean, who doesn't want to remember the time they rocked the pregnancy glow?

And why not involve the whole entourage? Drag your partner and loved ones into the frame, because nothing says "emotional and heartwarming" like coordinating outfits and forced smiles. "Yes, honey, we'll cherish this awkwardly posed photo forever!"

Week 24 – 6th month– 2nd Trymester!
Your baby

Your baby is growing like a little cob of corn in there!
Picture that tasty comparison as you enter the 24th week of pregnancy.
Your tiny superstar now tips the scale at over 500 grams and measures
around 20 centimeters from head to sitting position.
It's a growth spurt galore, and your baby is flexing those muscles!

Tiny Dancer: Your Baby's Dance Moves at 23 Weeks
Speaking of muscles, your baby's moves are turning into a full-blown
dance routine. Those kicks, squirms, and jigs in your belly are becoming
regular stars of the show. You might even notice patterns—maybe your
little one is a night owl with a penchant for evening performances. But just
like any star, they need their beauty rest too, so expect some quieter
moments when they're catching their Z's.

You might be wondering about the magic number of movements you
should feel at 24 weeks. Your doctor might introduce you to the "baby
movement monitoring" gig, asking you to count those little kicks and
wiggles at specific times of the day. It's like a backstage pass to your baby's
energetic routines.

Prepping for the Big Breath
Even though your baby's lungs are officially on the scene, they're
practicing their breathing game. The star of this show is called surfactant,
a substance that inflates those precious air sacs. They'll start producing
this superhero surfactant around the 26th week, getting all set for their big
performance outside the womb.

Now, let's talk ears!
Your baby's inner ear is making its grand entrance around this time. This
little marvel handles balance and orientation, helping your baby figure out
if they're doing a belly roll or a somersault in there.

Glowing and Growing

Your belly is expanding faster than your to-do list, and by the 24th week, you've gained a cool 4.5-7 kilograms of pregnancy glory. Embrace that beautiful bump, because it's all part of the amazing journey you're on.

Your Pregnancy Power Couple for a Comedy-Free Journey!

Keeping up with a balanced diet and regular exercise is like giving yourself a double dose of feel-good magic. Not only will you physically feel better, but your mental sparkle will shine even brighter. Plus, let's not forget the bonus points: staying active now can make shedding those extra pounds after the big "welcome to the world" moment a tad easier.

Backache Blues

Now, let's talk about those superhero sore backs. They might feel like unwelcome guests crashing the pregnancy party, but fear not! You've got options. Ever thought about rocking a pregnancy belt or a snazzy support band? These little helpers can give your abdomen the extra TLC it deserves, especially during your pregnancy gymnastics routine.

So there you have it: rocking that growing belly, supporting your body like the superstar you are, and keeping the good vibes flowing with nutritious nosh and a dose of those endorphins.
You've got this, pregnancy champ!

What's new this week?

Ah, the ever-changing canvas of pregnancy skin – a masterpiece painted with a palette of hormones and pigments. As you journey through the 24th week, your skin may embark on a symphony of transformations:

Stretch Mark Chronicles

Ah, the age-old saga of stretch marks. As your body expands and embraces its new form, these marks may sneak onto your canvas, particularly on the abdomen, buttocks, and breasts. While they can't be completely avoided, remember, they're your battle scars of transformation. Over time, they'll fade to delicate whispers, telling tales of your journey.

Pigment Play

Hormones turn skin cells into artistic virtuosos, unveiling darker spots on your face and body. It's like a natural paintbrush dipped in melanin is giving you freckles and chloasma (those facial sunspots). Don't fret, these temporary masterpieces often fade after birth. To keep your canvas clear, steer clear of heavy sun exposure and invite sunscreen as your protective muse.

The Itchy Quirk

As your canvas stretches, it might itch like a work-in-progress yearning for completion. Combat this sensation with the soothing strokes of moisturizing lotion. It's like giving your canvas a gentle caress to pacify its artistic aspirations.

Round Ligament Serenade

Ah, the harmonious strains of round ligament pain. It's like a symphony of discomfort that might play on one or both sides of your abdomen or hips. The ligaments holding your uterus in place are stretching and straining, creating this rather common tune. Stretch gently, shift positions, and maybe even do a little interpretive dance to ease the notes of discomfort. But if the melody crescendos into intense pain or is joined by fever or bleeding, let your doctor take the conductor's baton for an examination.

Slumber Sonata

Finding the perfect sleep position with your expanding belly can be like trying to compose the perfect sonata. Enter the pregnancy pillows, your orchestra of comfort. With a pillow between your knees and one under your belly, you'll drift into a dreamy nocturne, resting like a maestro on a cloud of support.

Balance Ballet

As your body transforms, its balance choreography changes too. Your center of gravity is a bit like a pirouetting dancer, sometimes making balance a delicate pas de deux. Dizziness might join the performance as your circulation pirouettes. Slow, graceful movements, hydrating like a hydration ballet, and a vigilant stance can keep your steps steady. And if dizziness steps onto the stage, rest like a prima ballerina – on your side. If questions arise about these dancing symptoms, let your doctor become the choreographer of advice.

The belly-bump conundrum!

As your pregnancy play reaches its 24-week intermission, you and your partner might be wondering about the safety of the romantic scenes.

But fret not, the safety script is simple: if your pregnancy is going according to plan, there's usually no backstage drama when it comes to intimacy.

However, if complications enter the stage left, temporary abstinence may be the director's call. Remember, every pregnancy plot is unique, so only your trusty pregnancy doctor can provide personalized advice.

And speaking of plot twists, your and your partner's desire for those romantic scenes might undergo a rewrite too.

The Glucose Load Test

Meanwhile, the glucose load test makes its cameo appearance between weeks 21 and 26, like a superhero swooping in to detect the possibility of gestational diabetes. But don't worry, this isn't a villainous plot – it's just a precautionary measure to ensure everything's on track.

The seat belt choreography!

As your "baby belly" takes center stage, the choreography of fastening your seat belt requires a tweak. The lap belt gets comfy under the belly, nestled against your hip bones. The shoulder belt? A true diva – it takes its place across your chest, not under your shoulder, ensuring a safe encore for both you and your budding star. Just remember, no part of that seat belt should play near your abdomen. Safety first – it's the golden rule for your pregnancy journey!

Hydration, the unsung hero of your pregnancy saga!

As you play the lead role in this incredible journey, don't forget to keep the hydration spotlight shining bright. Your baby-to-be is counting on those 8 to 12 glasses of fluid daily to support their grand debut.

Now, if you're battling forgetfulness amidst the hustle and bustle of your pregnancy production, fear not! Cue the dramatic entrance of reminders. Your trusty phone, with its periodic water cues, ensures you won't miss a sip.
Or, for the tech-savvy mom, there's the app option, ready to track and nudge your hydration routine. For an elegant touch, the starring role goes to the bottles of water, strategically placed like set decorations, ensuring you stay hydrated through each scene.

Labor Preferences – Your Personal Script for the Grand Finale!

The plot thickens as you cross the 24-week mark. It's like you've reached intermission, and now it's time to discuss the second act – labor preferences! Gather your partner, your supporting cast (which could include a friend or family member), and your provider for a backstage chat. Sharing your personal labor script ensures everyone's on the same page for the grand finale. Your partner, in a starring role, becomes your support superhero – alleviating pain, offering encouragement, and providing emotional comfort. This is the time to script your birth plan, to interview, and to ensure your dream labor performance takes center stage. The countdown is on, and you're the director of this incredible show!

The plot takes an intriguing twist

Your dreams become vivid tapestries, painted with colors and scenarios you never imagined. It's like your subconscious has joined the cast, producing a show of its own.
And focus? Well, that's taken a bow and wandered off stage. It's all part of the enigmatic "pregnancy amnesia" and intense dream phenomenon. Just remember, in this captivating journey, the unexpected is the norm!

Your baby

Your little one is rocking the "baby skin" look – still thin, delicate, and oh-so-pale. But guess what? This cutie is on a plumping-up spree!
Thanks to some baby magic involving fat pads and muscle growth, your munchkin is becoming rounder and more toddler-like every single day.
And the best part? There's a new hue in town – pink! Tiny blood vessels are throwing a colorful party under that skin, giving it a rosy touch.

Now, let's talk brainy stuff
Your baby's brain is like a VIP club with different sections. The cerebral cortex? It's got layers, and it's the happening spot for complex activities. But wait, there's more! Other brain areas are stealing the spotlight, for now, controlling the show like early achievers.

Oh, and here's a breath of fresh air – literally
In the baby workshop, the lungs are getting cozy with their new blood vessels, while the nostrils are opening up like curtains on a big stage.
All of this is like prep for that epic first breath your little star will take.
And speaking of vessels, they're not just chilling in the lungs – they're popping up under the skin too, making it all pink and fabulous.

Your body

Congratulations, your uterus is now the proud owner of a soccer ball-sized upgrade! Your little one's cozy home is expanding, and that might explain why your internal organs are doing a little shuffle for space.
Picture this: Your uterus, measuring about 25 centimeters from your pubic bone to that sweet spot halfway between your belly button and sternum, is giving your body a creative rearrangement!

Let's talk about the "glucose test."
It's like a pop quiz for your sugar levels, and it's usually scheduled between your 24th and 28th weeks of pregnancy.

This test is on a mission to uncover any potential signs of gestational diabetes. Don't worry, you're not alone – about two to five percent of moms-to-be get to be in this glucose-testing club.

It's like a little sugar adventure: first, you'll sip a sugar solution and then have your blood drawn a short while later to see how your body reacts. If your blood sugar levels are doing their own funky dance, no worries – it just means you'll have a follow-up test to see if gestational diabetes is hanging around.

If it's a positive result, don't worry, it's not the end of the world – just a small diet and lifestyle adjustment. Some might even call it a "sweet" way to keep things in balance! So, sip that sugar potion and let your body show off its glucose-handling skills.

What surprises might await you in week 25?

The UTI Dance Party – Why You Shouldn't Cha-Cha Along!
Pregnancy sometimes comes with surprise guests – like urinary tract infections (UTIs). So, if you've got the urge, make a beeline for the bathroom. If you sense a sizzle, sting, or an unwanted aroma while doing your business, it might be the UTI dance.
Don't just cha-cha along – give your doc a call pronto. Ignoring these unwelcome visitors isn't on the agenda, since UTIs during pregnancy can throw a not-so-fun party with serious consequences.

Things to consider

- Get ready for the glucose test to check for gestational diabetes.
- Keep an eye out for sneaky urinary tract infections – they're more common during pregnancy.
- Time to plan that maternity leave like a boss!

Buckle up for some serious baby milestones this week – it's like your little one is gearing up for the baby Olympics inside your belly!

I smell victory
Your baby's nostrils are making their debut, and they're not just for show. It's like the grand opening of the breathing practice studio, complete with newly developed lung muscles.
But wait, there's no air in there – so your baby's doing the "in and out" routine with the fetal waters. They're like the cutest little aquatic gymnasts, getting those breathing muscles in shape!

Aquatic Gymnastics
And speaking of gymnastics, your baby's got some serious reflexes. The sucking game is strong, so strong that when their hand swings by their face, they might just start sucking on their thumb or giving their fingers a taste test. It's like they're the world's tiniest food critic!

Get a grip, baby!
Now, let's talk about grip strength – your baby's basically in training to be the next weightlifting champion. That grip is so strong that even your newborn's handshake would probably put ours to shame. And their favorite workout equipment? The umbilical cord!
But no worries, that cord's built tough, like the superhero cape of the baby world.

Could those eyes lie?
And those eyes? Oh, they're getting ready for their big reveal too. While the iris has made its entrance, the color palette is still under construction. It's like they're setting up the color wheel for the most stunning eyes ever. So, if you're wondering what shade those peepers will be, the surprise is all part of the baby magic.

Culinary duo - your first teamwork

Get ready for some culinary teamwork, because your little sidekick is sharing your meal plan! It's like you're both in this delicious adventure together, creating a menu for the ultimate tag-team experience.

Listen up, Mama – keeping that blood sugar in check is your secret weapon. Think of it like your energy fuel gauge. If it dips too low, you might start feeling like you're doing a dizzy disco. Nobody wants that, right? So, embrace those small but frequent meals like mini power boosts. Your body's thanking you in advance for this snacking strategy!

And hey, if you're a spicy food warrior, don't worry, your spice passport is still valid! Your taste buds deserve some excitement, after all. But here's the thing – if you're about to dive into a culinary spicy adventure for the first time, take it slow. Your tummy might not be ready for that rollercoaster just yet.

So, get ready to be the ultimate mealtime duo, you and your tiny taste tester. From keeping the blood sugar dance in check to embarking on spicy food escapades, you're teaming up for a gastronomic journey like no other.

Bon appétit, mama-to-be!

Any new symptoms?

Nope, none, nada... no changes... Not the best news, but hey... at least no new adventures to add.

Things to consider

Here's the secret weapon

Those little snacks - mini-munchies of energy. Stock up on goodies like fruit or yogurt – they're like the sidekicks that keep your body fueled throughout the day. It's like you're creating your own snack oasis, ready to tackle any hunger pangs that come your way.

Week 27 – 7th month– 3rd Trymester!
Your baby

Guess what? Our little speed racer is on the move! Though still a work in progress, this baby's brain and lungs are like those last-minute party planners trying to get things sorted.

No worries, though – there's a solid 13-week boot camp before the grand entrance into the world. Talk about a deadline!

Baby's Big Reveal: Eyelids Unveil the Baby Cinema!
Hold onto your hats, folks – those baby eyelids, closed for what feels like an eternity (well, four months in baby time), are finally ready to reveal the world. It's like the curtains are lifting on the tiniest Broadway show, starring your baby!
The brain's got the spotlight on vision, and those peepers are all in for the show. Lights, shadows, and all the fascinating things the world has to offer – welcome to the baby cinema!

Baby's Belly Dance Extravaganza: Rock and Roll in the Womb!
Oh, and who needs a fancy hammock when you've got a belly? This little one's sleeping technique is a full-on dance party. With every gentle jiggle of your everyday errands, this baby's cozy as can be, swaying like they're at a concert. Thanks, Amniotic Waters – you're the original rock and roll!

Mini Food Critic in the Making: Spicy Taste Tests and Hiccup Symphonies!
Hold on to your taste buds, because this baby's got 'em! They're basically a mini food critic in there, discerning the daily menu of amniotic fluid. You know how they say babies inherit their parents' traits? Well, your baby might be inheriting your love for spicy food too. Cue the mini fiesta or the hiccup symphony – it's all part of the spicy taste test!

So, buckle up, because this little wonder is getting ready to join the world with a flair for drama (curtain call!), a knack for rhythm (rock on!), and a sophisticated palate (spicy dance party!).

Life's about to get a whole lot more entertaining – for you and the baby!

Breast Fashion Makeover: The Nipple Halo Chronicles!
Hold onto your hats, ladies, because your breasts are on a wild journey of their own during and after pregnancy! You might have already noticed that your breast's "nipple halo" (sounds almost heavenly, right?) is putting on a show of its own. It's like your breasts are having their own fashion makeover!

When Skin Borders Go Rogue!
In the early stages, those halos decided to darken up a bit – think of it as their mysterious, moody phase. But oh, they weren't satisfied with just that! As time goes on, that darker skin might go beyond the traditional halo borders and spread like an adventurous explorer, claiming new territory on your breast canvas. It's like they're trying on a new accessory that covers up to half the breast – very avant-garde!

Sci-Fi Boobies
Now, before you start wondering if your breasts are auditioning for a role in a sci-fi movie, rest assured that this is all part of the grand transformation. Your breasts are just painting temporary masterpieces that will likely start to retreat before your little one hits their first birthday.

How you might feel this week?

Where Salvador Dalí Would Applaud!
Get ready to dive into the wildest dream circus of your life – because if you're riding the pregnancy train, your dreams are putting on a show that'd make Broadway jealous! We're talking dreams that would make Salvador Dalí do a double take and Shakespeare give you a standing ovation.

Turning Nightly Fantasies into Epics!
Blame it on those hormone rockstars that are throwing a party in your body, waving their hormonal batons and making your dreams go from zero to surreal in seconds. It's like your brain's creative department is working overtime, churning out plots and characters that even Hollywood scriptwriters would envy.

Where Drama Meets Comedy!

Let's not forget about the emotional roller coaster you're on. Your mind's got its own VIP section for dealing with all those thoughts and feelings – and it's called the dream realm. It's like your dreams are the canvas for your mind's masterpiece, where it splashes colors of drama, comedy, and everything in between.

Who Needs Netflix Anyway?

If you find yourself starring in a dream where you're sipping tea with a talking elephant while riding a rainbow roller coaster – don't worry, you're not alone. It's just your body's way of processing the fantastic journey you're on. Who needs Netflix when you've got your own dream theater, right?

Things to consider

Doula: Your Birth's Fairy Godparent and Emotional MVP!

All right, let's talk about having your very own birth MVP – a doula! Picture this: you're about to step onto the grand stage of childbirth, and in walks your emotional cheerleader, your birth BFF, your doula. They're like the fairy godparent of labor, armed with a toolkit of emotional support and expert guidance.

Imagine having someone by your side who's not just holding your hand, but holding space for your feelings, fears, and hopes. A doula is like that wise friend who's been through it all before and knows the secret codes to soothing your nerves and boosting your confidence.

They're not here to deliver the baby – leave that to the professionals – but they're here to deliver something just as important: reassurance, encouragement, and a shoulder to lean on. From massaging away tension to whispering words of encouragement, they've got all the tricks up their sleeves.

So, if you're pondering whether to welcome a doula into your birth dream team, think of it as inviting the ultimate emotional lifeguard to your pool of labor waters. With a doula in your corner, you're not just facing childbirth, you're conquering it with a sidekick who's got your back no matter what twists and turns the journey takes.

Week 28 – 7th month – 3rd Trymester!
Your baby

Light show time!
Your little star is really getting into the groove. Last week, those eyes popped open for the first peek. And now, if you play spotlight with a bright light on your belly, your baby might just open those peepers and do a little turn-away dance. It's like their own mini disco!

Sound asleep?
Nah, your baby's brain is rocking to the beat of the outside world. Those brainwaves are tuning into sounds around them, and even their sleep patterns are starting to groove. As you get closer to the big day, their sleep routine will become a real headliner.

Time for some lung action!
Your baby's little lungs are gearing up for showtime. Soon enough, that first inhale will send oxygen coursing through those tiny blood vessels, making your baby a breathing superstar. And guess what? Their body is cooking up a special surfactant that keeps the air bubbles from sticking together, so they'll be ready to rock those breaths post-birth. Their bronchi are also working overtime, branching out into a full lung symphony.

Star-studded eyes!
Those baby blues (or browns or greens) are getting more active. Your baby's eyes are cracking open, and they might even throw in a blink for good measure. And hey, shine a flashlight near that belly stage, and your little rockstar might give you a kick in return. It's like they're jamming along with the light show!

Your body

Spotting some battle scars?
Don't sweat it, mama! Those stretch marks are like badges of honor, proof of the incredible journey your body's been on. While you can't exactly kick them out of the party, you can definitely make them feel less prominent.

Keep your weight gain in check, rock a nourishing diet, stay hydrated like a boss, groove to some exercise tunes, and treat your skin to some silky cream. Dry or itchy vibes? Not on our watch!

Here's the sweet part: after the pregnancy curtain falls, those marks take a chill pill. They'll change from bold red to a sleek silvery hue, like your body's own special art installation. So go ahead, wear those stripes with pride!

Possible symptoms awaiting you

Pregnancy Picasso time!
As your journey unfolds, you might notice some stretch marks making a guest appearance on your abdomen, breasts, hips, and thighs. Let's be real, these little lines are like nature's doodles on your canvas. While the consensus is that dodging them is a bit like trying to dodge raindrops, slathering on a cream or oil might give them a bit of a gentle nudge.

Mom's Gift of Customized Masterpieces!
Genetics could be holding the crayons on this one – if your mom had her own set of marks, you might just be getting your own customized masterpiece. But here's the silver lining: post-pregnancy, these lines usually decide to take a chill pill and fade a bit.
So don't stress, Mama, you're a work of art in progress!

Coordination Mishaps: When Pregnancy Turns You into a Dance-Off Pro!
Speaking of progress, your coordination might decide to take a vacation right about now. Blame it on that shifting center of gravity and those oh-so-relaxed joints. Suddenly, you might find yourself having a dance-off with tables or tripping over your own toes.
The trick?
Slow down, slip into some comfy flats, and move at a pace that gives your wobbly moments a chance to shine.

Rh factor rendezvous

If the lab report dances to the tune of Rh(-) for you, it's time for a safety measure. This week, you'll be treated to an anti-D injection just in case your baby's playlist is more Rh(+). This backstage move prevents any potential antibodies from crashing the party in your bloodstream. Your little one's Rh factor will get its solo debut after birth, and if it's a positive hit, you'll get an encore of the anti-D injection to keep the harmony for future gigs.

Bid adieu to heels

The catwalk may have to wait because your graceful glide might turn into a tumble with those high heels. Thanks to your shifting center of gravity and your body's newfound talent for wobbles, flats might become your new BFF. It's a sensible choice that saves you from some not-so-sensible stumbles.

VIP guest list for delivery day

Time to play casting director for your delivery room performance! Think about who you want to share the spotlight with when the big moment arrives. Whether it's your partner, a doula, or a certain grandma-to-be, it's your call. Choose the support squad that vibes with your birth-day vision.

Cute Enough to Melt Your Heart!

Guess who's getting their adorable game face on? That's right, your tiny superstar is gearing up to rock the "fully developed baby" look! Those once-squishy features are shaping up into the cutest bundle of joy you've ever laid eyes on. It's like watching a masterpiece come to life, one chubby cheek at a time.

Your Baby's Neural Network Unveiled!

And speaking of masterpieces, your baby's brain is putting on quite the show. Not only can it handle some serious temperature control, but it's also flexing its impressive nerve cell collection – we're talking hundreds of billions! It's like your baby's brain is setting up a neural network that's ready to power them through all the adventures life has in store.

But hold onto your baby blankets, because here's a fun fact: your little Picasso won't be producing any more of these fancy nerve cells post-birth. It's like they're wrapping up their masterpiece before the big gallery reveal!

Fashion-Forward Baby Skin

Let's not forget about that adorable baby skin. It's smoother and paler, thanks to all the dedicated weight gain efforts. Think of it as your baby's own fashion statement – paler and smoother, just in time for the grand debut. And guess what? All that precious baby fat they're accumulating? It's like nature's own cozy sweater, keeping them warm and snuggly.

So, get ready to meet your soon-to-be heart-stealer, with a brain that's wired for greatness, skin that's ready for the spotlight, and a physique that's prepped for endless cuddles. Your little one's got it all, and they're ready to shine!

Whoa, it's getting cozy in that baby bungalow!

Your little VIP guest has gone and taken up most of the space in their plush uterine suite. It's like they're the star of their very own real estate show, turning every corner into prime baby space.

Baby Tetris

Your baby is basically playing the ultimate game of baby Tetris in there. With around 10 weeks left on their lease, about 96% of these tiny tenants are choosing the head-down position for the grand move-out day. They're getting ready to make their big entrance like the VIPs they are!

Belly Dance Party

Now, let's talk about the rock concert happening inside your belly. With all that real estate taken up, your baby's got some serious moves to show off. It's like they've turned your belly into a dance floor, complete with kicks, jabs, and even a little elbow and knee action. They're grooving like there's no tomorrow, giving you a taste of the party that's about to hit the outside world.

You and Baby on a Pounds-Packing Journey!

Get ready for the ultimate tag team weight gain championship – you and your baby are about to be on the same journey for the next three months! It's like you've both signed up for the "Let's Pack on the Pounds" challenge.

Picture this: your baby is gearing up for their grand entrance by putting on some adorable baby chub. And guess what? You're on the same track! As your little one gets ready to shine, you can expect to team up with them and add around 5 kg to your weight during this final trimester.

It's like you and your baby are partnering up for this last leg of the pregnancy marathon, both working to ensure that your little one has all the snuggly padding they need for their big debut.
It's a journey of growth, nourishment, and teamwork – you're literally growing together!

Oh, the joys of pregnancy – leg cramps decided to join the party!
It's like your legs are putting on a secret dance performance, complete with unexpected twists and turns.
Now, here's the funny thing: even the experts are having a little debate about what exactly causes these cramps. Some think it's like your legs are doing a superhero workout to handle the extra load you're carrying around. Others suspect it's a calcium or potassium craving – your legs might be on the hunt for some serious nutrients.

And let's not forget about the mysterious uterus magician! This little superstar might be playing a part in the leg cramp symphony by giving your nerves a gentle squeeze. It's like your uterus has a secret talent for choreography, and your legs are the unwitting stars of the show.

So, how do you tackle these surprise dance routines? Imagine you're teaching your legs some yoga moves – gently stretch them by bending your foot and pulling those toes back towards you. It's like you're showing your legs some post-cramp self-care, giving them a little stretchy TLC.

But hey, prevention's the name of the game too!
Flex those stretching muscles throughout the day especially before you hit the dreamland stage. And don't forget your nutrient buddies – calcium and potassium. Load up on foods that have these two on the guest list, and your legs might just thank you with fewer surprise performances.

So, remember, you're not alone in this dance battle with your legs. With a little stretchy magic and some nutrient power, you're ready to show those leg cramps who's boss.
Keep on dancing, mama-to-be!

Things to consider

Let's give a standing ovation to the power of nutrients!
Load up on meals that are bursting with calcium and potassium, and your body might just be singing "thank you" instead of cramp-filled ballads. It's like you're treating your body to a nutrient-packed symphony, making sure everything's in harmony.

Baby's Brain: Getting Wrinklier and Wiser!"

Hold onto your hats, because your baby's brain is getting a makeover! There's a whole lotta progress happening in that noggin of theirs. This week, their brain starts taking on a cool, crinkly look – kind of like a textured masterpiece. These groovy textures are called brain ganglia, and they're like the brain's way of saying, "Bring on the cells!" These wrinkles give the brain more room to welcome new cells.
Talk about brain power!

Baby's Fine Fur Is Packing Its Bags

Your baby's development is in turbo mode. And guess what? The brain's not the only thing evolving – that ultra-fine mess called lanugo that once cozied up on your baby is now packing its bags and preparing to leave.

Calcium Construction Crew

Baby's building bones and calcium's like the construction worker in the hard hat.

Baby's Nutritional Allies for a Strong Start!

Iron's on the scene, too, courtesy of prenatal vitamins and your element-rich eats. This iron stash is all prepped to keep your little one nourished for the first six to nine months of their journey. And the protein posse? They're here to support the development of cells throughout your baby's whole body.

Your body

Weight gain alert!

Your baby's going for gold in the weight gain department, with a double or even triple feat lined up in the weeks ahead.
And here's a little secret: You'll also be stepping up your own weight gain game during this time. Teamwork at its finest!

Itchy Times

Ah, the seventh month's special feature: itchiness. Blame it on that skin stretching like a champion on your growing belly. But here's the deal – scratching's not the solution. Instead, give your belly some love with gentle massages using a moisturizing lotion. Your skin will thank you for the TLC!

The unexpected guests that nobody invited!

These pesky little things are like the party crashers of your prenatal experience. Blame it on the increased pressure down there or those hormones that seem to be throwing a never-ending party in your body. So, picture this: your rear end is hosting its exclusive soiree, complete with swollen, painful guests who just won't leave. They're like the rowdy neighbors in the apartment upstairs, making your life a bit more interesting (read: uncomfortable).

To kick these uninvited visitors out, you might want to consider some dietary changes – think of it as a menu makeover for your derriere. Fiber-rich foods and lots of water, like the bouncers at the door, can help keep things moving smoothly and show those hemorrhoids to the exit.

To tackle the pesky problem of hemorrhoids, you've got a few home remedies up your sleeve that are as classic as your grandma's secret cookie recipe:

The Soothing Soak: Imagine this - a mini spa day for your derriere. Fill your bathtub with lukewarm water (around 40 degrees Celsius) to a depth of about 10 centimeters. Now, add some herbal magic like oak bark, chamomile, or a blend of sage and chestnut bark. Take a seat, keep your legs bent, and relax for a maximum of 10 minutes. It's like a calm oasis in the middle of your day!

The Cool Compress: Think of it as the ice pack's classy cousin. Wrap an ice cube in a soft cloth and apply it gently to those sore spots. If you're feeling adventurous, you can even make a supercool tampon with onion juice and a dash of olive oil. And guess what? Black tea isn't just for sipping - a damp tea bag can also work wonders as a poultice.

The Warm Bath: It's time to give your "little" behind a warm embrace. Fill your bathtub with warm water and add a few drops of soothing oils like lavender, rosemary, or lemon. This isn't just relaxation time; it's also promoting better blood flow and reducing those pesky swellings.

The Creamy Heroes: When your at-home magic tricks don't quite cut it, don't worry; you've got reinforcements. Head to your friendly neighborhood pharmacy for some suppositories or ointments specially crafted for this situation. They're like the superheroes of hemorrhoid relief.

Remember, you've got a range of remedies to try, and if one doesn't quite do the trick, don't be afraid to explore others. Your comfort is the name of the game, and these home remedies are here to help you score big in the comfort department.

Things to consider

Nourish Wisely

Your baby's got a growth spurt agenda, and that means loading up on calcium, iron, and protein. These nutrients are like the VIPs of the baby development party, so make sure your meals are packed with these powerhouses.

Birthing School Bonanza

Ready for some birthing school action? Time to flex those muscles, both physically and mentally. Those recommended exercises? It's like a dress rehearsal for the big day.

Get your groove on and be prepared for the journey ahead.

Doctor Detective

The quest for the right doctor begins! It's like assembling your dream team for your baby's journey. Whether it's a pediatrician, family doctor, or nurse practitioner, the search begins now.

Don't be shy – start early and ask friends for recommendations. This is your baby's healthcare partner, so take your time, check out your options, and find the one who vibes with your family's needs.

After all, this is a relationship that'll last through the first year of your baby's life and beyond!

Week 31 – 7th month– 3rd Trymester!

Your baby

Hold onto your excitement, because your baby's gearing up for some incredible changes this month! Just picture it – they've been in this cozy curled-up position for a while now, like a little adventurer getting ready to set foot in a new world.

Growing Strong

Your baby's like a superstar athlete, gaining about an extra kilogram of body weight this month. It's like they're bulking up for their big debut, getting stronger and more ready to face the world with you in just nine weeks.

Thumbelina

Imagine this adorable scenario – your baby, cozy as can be, suddenly feels a hand near their face. They might do a little head dance, like they're on a mission to find their thumb and give it a taste test. It's like their seeking reflex is a treasure hunt for that tiny thumb, a sneak peek into their natural instinct to grasp and suck after birth.

Your body

Everest, here I come!

Hey there, Mama, feeling like you're climbing Everest just to catch a breath? Your expanding uterus is like the star of the show, pushing your diaphragm right up against your lungs.

Now, here's a silver lining for you – if your baby's chilling out low in your belly, consider yourself in the lucky club. Those high-belly moms have it a bit tougher like their diaphragms are doing a limbo dance. But don't worry, you've got a secret weapon: deep breaths and a little slow-down time. It's like giving your body a chance to catch its breath, quite literally.

Imagine this: as you're reaching that 37th or 38th week, it's like your baby's deciding to take the elevator to a lower floor. And guess what? It's like the grand release for your lungs and diaphragm. Breathing gets a little easier, and you're feeling like a true oxygen superstar.

Braxton Hicks or the Real Deal? Your Contractions Decoded!
From the second trimester's middle to the third trimester's start, you're in the lookout mode. Preterm labor or Braxton Hicks contractions?
Here's the tip: if they're irregular and give you a break when you switch things up or take a stroll, they're like the friendly "hello" of Braxton Hicks contractions. Not a cause for alarm, just your body practicing for the big day.

Things to consider

Get ready to play the ultimate matchmaker – it's like finding the perfect puzzle piece for your baby's care! Whether it's a nanny, daycare, or a loving relative, the time to start exploring your options is now.

Care Hunt Begins
It's like embarking on a care adventure for your little one. Whether you're dreaming of a nanny, checking out daycares, or thinking about that extra special relative, now's the moment to dive in. It's like crafting the best environment for your baby's growth and happiness.

Interview Extravaganza
Imagine this – you're like a casting director, interviewing potential caregivers for your baby's star role. It's a chance to find the perfect fit, someone who shares your vision for your baby's care journey. So, get those questions ready and embrace the role of the ultimate interviewer!

Sitter Squad
Picture this – you might not need full-time care, but you're gathering your dream team of babysitters for those special occasions. It's like building a squad of backup heroes, ready to step in when you need a helping hand or a well-deserved break.

Week 32 – 8th month– 3rd Trymester!
Your baby

Guess who's playing musical chairs in there? Your baby!
By this week, they're likely doing a little dance routine, trying to find the perfect seat for their grand entrance.

Position Switcheroo
It's like a baby ballet of positioning – most little ones are all about that head-down vibe now. This is the golden position, the one where they're like, "Yep, this is where I want to be when the curtain rises." But hey, don't be surprised if they're feeling a little adventurous. Changing positions a few times is totally their style.

Amniotic Adventures
Imagine your baby swimming in their personal pool of about 0.95 liters of amniotic fluid. It's like they're in their very own aquatic playground, and with that much fluid, changing positions isn't too tough. They're like the ultimate synchronized swimmer, gracefully gliding from one pose to another.

Skin Smoothness
Your baby's like a little superstar with a smooth, pink skin glow – all thanks to that adorable fatty tissue. It's like they're getting ready for their big close-up, and they're looking as dreamy as ever.

Your body

Your Pregnancy Journey: From Tiny Uterus to Neighborhood Takeover!
Your baby's home sweet home, the uterus, has gone through a massive glow-up, expanding around 500 times its initial size since the pregnancy kicked off. It's like a real estate market boom in there!
This growth spurt is so impressive that it's almost taken over the entire abdominal neighborhood.

But, here's the thing - this growth spurt comes with some unintended consequences. Your internal organs, those poor roommates in this cozy uterine apartment, are getting nudged around, leading to some digestive discomfort. It's like a cramped elevator ride during rush hour.

And guess what? The uterus isn't just stopping at the abdominal border; it's reaching for the stars. Well, almost. The lower part is cozying up to your ribs, and the upper section is having a friendly chat with your diaphragm. This can make taking a deep breath feel like a marathon.

But wait, there's more!
Your belly is like the ultimate storage unit right now. It's housing not only your precious little one but also a bunch of amniotic fluid, the trusty placenta, and a ton of extra blood and water. All of this adds up to around 6-7 kilograms of extra weight for you. It's like carrying around a small suitcase everywhere you go. But hey, it's all part of the magical journey of pregnancy!

Possible symptoms this week

When the Tiny Dancer Gets Too Enthusiastic
Ah, the joys of baby's movements – it's like your little one's having a dance party in there! But hold on, there might be a footloose moment that's not exactly pleasant like a tiny dancer getting a bit too enthusiastic under your chest.

Fear not, Mama, you've got moves of your own!
If you find yourself in a foot traffic jam, consider a little side-to-side action. Lying on your side or changing positions is like giving your baby a gentle nudge on the dance floor. It's an invitation for them to shift their moves and find a more comfortable spot.

Things to consider

Welcome to the double-check phase, mama – it's like your pregnancy is getting a VIP upgrade! Once you hit week 32, your doctor's going to be your partner in making sure everything's sailing smoothly.

Doctor Duo

Get ready for the dynamic doctor duo – now it's every two weeks for those check-ups. They're like your pregnancy superheroes, on the lookout for any potential hiccups like infections, signs of premature labor, or pre-eclampsia. It's like having a top-notch security detail for you and your baby.

Hospital Recon

Time to get to know your baby's future debut spot! A visit to the hospital where you'll be giving birth is like a backstage tour before the big show. You'll get to see the labor rooms, check out the postpartum care setup, and understand the ins and outs of procedures and registration. It's like having the ultimate pre-show backstage pass, so when the curtain rises, you're ready to rock and roll.

Childbirth Pro

It's like going back to school, but this time it's all about childbirth. Those classes are like your crash course in baby delivery – ask questions, share hopes and fears, and be a sponge for all that knowledge.
Don't forget to bring your partner along for the ride!
They're your trusty sidekick, and together, you're becoming the ultimate dream team for the big moment.

Week 33 – 8th month– 3rd Trymester!
Your baby

Baby's got senses on overdrive!
Your little champ is soaking in the underwater wonderland, wiggling toes and giving that thumb a taste test. Plus, the amniotic fluid is like a tiny flavor party, and your heartbeat is like their personal lullaby.

Brainy business
The noggin is on a roll, growing the circumference by around 1.3 cm in just a week. Talk about brain gains!

Time to be the nutrition superhero!
Your baby's craving protein and fat like never before. So keep that balanced diet going strong. Right now, your cutie measures around 42 centimeters and tips the scales at about 2 kilograms.
But hang on – they're gearing up to double that weight in the next seven weeks!

Your body

When Your Belly Becomes a Dance Floor!
Wow, your little one is really making its presence known in there! With all that growth, it's no wonder there's less room for the amniotic fluid and more for your baby's kicks and punches.
Get ready for some lively dance moves from your tiny dancer!
And guess what?
You've got some sweet moves to soothe your little performer too! You can take a relaxing rock in a comfy rocking chair, bust a move on a pregnancy ball, or even try a little pelvic swaying in the hands and knees position. It's like a little dance party for two, where you're the DJ and your baby's the star!

Embrace the weight gain!
Your body is doing an amazing job of adding about 0.45 kilograms per week to nurture that growing bundle of joy. No need to hit the brakes on this weight gain journey – your little one is happily taking up space and needs those extra pounds for their grand entrance. So, go ahead and enjoy this weighty adventure without worries. There's a whole post-delivery world for any weight-related thoughts later on!

Wrestling with wrist discomfort? You're not alone!
Carpal tunnel syndrome can join the pregnancy party, causing some swelling around your wrist nerves due to fluid retention. But don't fret – this unwelcome guest usually checks out after childbirth. In the meantime, consider switching up your sleep positions to give your hands and wrists a break. You might even become besties with a wrist brace to help keep things comfy. And of course, make sure to keep your doctor in the loop about any pains – they're there to help you navigate this wristy situation!

Things to consider

Nourish yourself right
Load up on protein and those good-for-you fats to keep you and your little one in tip-top shape!

Hospital-bound?
Time to put on your detective hat and check out the best route to get there. Planning ahead will make that journey smoother when the big day arrives!

Wrist action
If your wrists are staging a protest, consider donning a trusty wrist brace or getting creative with your sleep setup. Those z's and comfy wrists are a winning combo!

Your baby

Guess who's getting cozy in there? Your little one!
As the space starts to feel a bit snug, their movements might slow down a bit. It's like they're finding their comfy corner in their tiny abode.

Space Odyssey

Imagine your baby's like a little astronaut in their spaceship – the limited space is like their cue to take it easy on the acrobatics. Their movements might become more gentle, like a soft symphony playing in the background.

Chassis Update

If you're expecting a baby boy, guess what's happening? It's like the testicles are setting up shop in the scrotum, getting ready for the big debut. And here's a heads-up – if you notice the scrotum looking a bit bigger at birth, no worries! It's just a bit of fluid play, and it'll fade away like a fading star.

Blue-Eyed Wonder

Your baby's like a little mystery with blue eyes – it's like they've got their own unique shade ready for their debut. But wait, there's a twist! The full iris pigmentation process is like a gradual masterpiece. It's like their eyes are saying, "I'll reveal my true color once I've soaked in some light after birth!"

Slow-and-Steady Gain

Imagine your baby's like a master of the growth game, and they're slowing things down a bit. The weight gain is like a roller coaster easing into a gentle ride, getting ready for its grand appearance. And here's a fun thought – if they kept growing at this pace, they'd be a hefty 90 kg on their first birthday.
Now that's one big birthday bash!

It's like preparing for the final exam, where you're the star student and labor signs are your study material.

Contractions Calling

Imagine contractions are like little messengers, knocking on your door with news of the big day. When they show up, like clockwork, with intervals getting shorter and shorter, it's like the countdown has officially begun.

Sacrum Sensations

Picture this – your sacrum's like the backstage whisperer, giving you a heads-up. If you're feeling pain in that area, and it's hanging out with menstrual-like cramps, it's like a gentle tap on your shoulder saying, "Get ready, mama!"

Waters on the Move

Imagine your baby's like a little adventurer packing their bags. If you experience a "departure" of fetal waters, like a little rupture of the amniotic sac, it's like they're sending their RSVP for the big party. And don't forget the color – blood-colored leakage is like the red carpet, indicating that your cervix is getting in on the action too.

Early Birds

Signs of labor might decide to show up fashionably early, like a sneak peek of the grand show. It's like they're giving you a preview of the magic to come, days or even weeks before the actual big moment.

Remember, Mama, you're the conductor of this symphony, and your body's giving you cues like a melody leading up to the crescendo.
If any of these signs make an appearance, it's like your cue to call your doctor ASAP.

You're all set for this lesson in labor readiness – get ready to ace the ultimate test of motherhood!

Week 35 – 8th month– 3rd Trymester!
Your baby

Baby's Building Blocks: Growing Strong Inside the Belly!
At this point in the pregnancy journey, your little bundle of joy tips the scales at a cool 2 kilograms and stretches out to about 40 centimeters long. It's like having a precious watermelon-sized guest inside your belly.

Ultrasound Sneak Peek: Baby's Dress Rehearsal!
During those 35 weeks on the inside, your baby isn't just lounging around; they're putting on a show! You might catch them in action on an ultrasound, perhaps having a thumb-sucking session or practicing other moves for their big debut.

Baby's Weekly Weightlifting and Immunity Boost!
Speaking of practice, they're also beefing up their baby's body, gaining about 150-200 grams each week. It's like a mini-bulk-up session in there! But here's the superhero part: your baby is still getting a dose of antibodies through that trusty umbilical cord. It's like mom's special immunity delivery service, arming your little one with protective shields against future infections.
Talk about having a head start in life!

Baby's Lung Development: Preparing for the Grand Debut!
Those tiny lungs may be all set, but they're not quite ready for the grand opening outside the cozy womb. Premature babies can sometimes face a challenge called respiratory distress syndrome (RDS) if they arrive too early. So, your baby's gearing up for a smooth entrance into the world in the coming weeks!

Baby's Position: A puzzle piece falling into place
The ideal position for delivery is when your baby's head is down, facing your spine.
But wait, there's a plot twist! If your baby's bottom decides to make an entrance first, it's a "buttock delivery."
And guess what? Even in the cozy confines of your uterus, your little acrobat might still have some spins and turns left before the grand debut.

Iron Reserves: Your baby's building an iron stash,
Guess where they're getting it from? You! That's right, they're absorbing it from your body. So, roll out the iron-rich red carpet for the last trimester. Think leafy greens, legumes, and other iron-packed foods.
It's like giving your baby a nutritional power boost before the big day.

Position Changes: Heads or tails, baby's got options!
Just because they're in a certain position now doesn't mean they're locked in for delivery day. That little acrobat might flip and twirl a few times before the curtain call. It's like a preview of the star performance coming soon.

Baby's First Manicure: Get ready for some adorable baby nail action!
Those tiny fingers and toes have been growing their mini-masterpieces – the nails. You might even catch a glimpse of those little nails peeking out. It's like a baby's first postpartum manicure session, all ready for the world to see.

Your body

ABCS of GBS:
As you journey towards the 37th week, a new character might enter the story – Group B Streptococcus (GBS). Don't let the name intimidate you – it's harmless to you but could cause a hiccup during delivery for your little one.
Here's the script:

Testing Time: Your doctor might want to run a test to see if GBS is hanging around. It's a simple swab – from your vagina or rectum, or perhaps a urine sample. Think of it as a backstage pass to make sure everything's smooth for the main event.

The Role of GBS: GBS isn't causing any trouble for you, but it's a potential party crasher for your baby. If it decides to show up during delivery, it could lead to an infection. But don't worry – you're the star here, and there's a plan in place.

The Antibiotic Solution: If the test reveals you're in the GBS club, you've got a superhero – antibiotics. They'll be delivered intravenously (that's a fancy term for through a syringe into a vein in your arm) during labor and delivery. It's like a protective shield for your baby's grand entrance.

Baby Bump Reaches for the Stars: The Ribcage Rumble

In this stage of your pregnancy, your baby bump has taken center stage, and it's reaching for the stars, or at least your ribcage! Thanks to the generous amount of amniotic fluid, your diaphragm and stomach are practically rubbing elbows, which can lead to some not-so-fun pregnancy discomfort. It's like they're having a friendly neighborhood squabble in there.

Your uterus has been on the rise, and now it's positioned way up high, right under your ribcage arches. No wonder you might be feeling some added pressure on those ribs.

But here's a twist in the plot: those irregular contractions you're feeling aren't just for show. They're like the prelude to the grand finale, signaling that your little one's debut is on the horizon. These contractions might have made their debut around week 20, but with each passing week, they're getting more and more convincing, making your belly feel like a rock star, or at least, rock-solid.

Worth checking with your doc

Pain Medication Chat

Let's talk about comfort during labor – it's like your VIP pass to a smoother journey. Time to sit down with your doctor and have a heart-to-heart about pain medications. Whether you're into the idea of relief through an epidural, laughing gas, or other options, your doctor's like the expert tour guide through this realm. So open up the conversation and explore the choices that'll make your labor experience as comfortable as can be.

Cesarean Section Insights

Picture this – a different path to bringing your little one into the world. A cesarean section (C-section) is like the alternate route. It's when the baby comes into the spotlight through a surgical incision in your uterus and abdomen. But here's the deal – it's not the main route for most pregnancies. If you're curious, talk to your doctor about the circumstances that might lead to a C-section and when it could be on the table.

Your doctor is like the navigator on this journey, steering you through the possibilities.

Week 36 – 9th month–last moments :)
Your baby

Get ready for some fascinating baby facts that'll warm your heart and blow your mind!
Your baby's world is a captivating one, full of amazing discoveries.

Sweet Melodies

Picture this – your newborn is already a music critic! Studies have unveiled that they have a soft spot for their number one fan: YOU. That's right, your baby prefers the sound of your voice over all the other chatter in the world.

And guess what? They've got a memory like a jukebox too. If they've heard a song on repeat during their cozy womb days, they'll recognize and love it after they make their big debut.

Baby's First Playlist

Your baby's musical journey starts before birth! Pick a special time each day to play that favorite CD, sing that beloved song, or even read a story to your little one. It's like you're curating their first playlist – a mixtape of memories that'll stay with them forever.

Skull Secrets

Your baby's got a head start in the skull department! Those cranial bones are designed to be flexible, allowing for a smoother journey through the cervix and pelvis during birth. It's like nature's way of giving them a comfortable road trip without any bumps.

Ready, Set, Go...Almost

Get ready for a fun fact – your baby's got a well-equipped body! All systems are a go, except one – digestion. Since your baby's been getting their gourmet meals delivered via the umbilical cord, their stomach and intestines haven't clocked in for work yet. But don't worry, they're like culinary superstars ready to make their grand entrance within months of birth.

Hold onto your hats, because your uterus is like a real estate mogul, expanding to epic proportions! Imagine this: It's now a whopping thousand times larger than when it all started. It's like your baby's luxury penthouse, complete with room to stretch and grow.

The Final Act of Weight Gain: The Weighty Curtain Call

Now, let's talk numbers. You've been carrying around an extra load – about 11 to 13.5 kilograms of it. But here's the plot twist: the weight gain isn't done yet. Over the next four weeks, you might just add one or two more kilos to the mix. But here's the kicker – many women don't gain any weight at all during that last month of pregnancy. It's like the weight gain curtain call, with your body putting on a show of its own.

Pregnancy: When Your Ankles Join the Water Balloon Festival

And speaking of size, let's talk edema – that's the fancy term for fluid-related swelling. Even if it hasn't been an issue for you until now, the last month might bring a little extra fluid party to your body. It's like your body's throwing a hydration bash, and everyone's invited!

How you might feel in the week 36?

Hey there, mom-to-be, it's time for your weekly check-in with the doctor – and the countdown is officially on! Starting at week 36, your doctor's your partner in making sure this grand finale goes off without a hitch.

Doctor Dates

Get ready to be besties with your doctor, because you'll be seeing them every week now. They're like your pregnancy quarterback, making sure everything's in tip-top shape. Among other things, they'll be keeping an eagle eye on your blood pressure and checking for any sneaky proteins in your urine.

These little tests are like their detective tools, helping them keep pre-eclampsia at bay – that's the potential troublemaker that we're determined to keep out of the picture.

Rest and Rise

Treat yourself to a little relaxation oasis, mama. Whether it's elevating those feet like a relaxation pro or giving your left side some quality time – both positions are like a gentle massage for your circulation. Remember, staying hydrated is your best friend. Eight glasses of water a day might seem like a lot, but it's like the ultimate detox strategy, flushing out toxins, and keeping your blood volume in check.

Braxton-Hicks Bootcamp

Think of these contractions as your body's warm-up routine for the big event. They're like a little practice session, getting your uterus ready for the main act. But here's the twist – they're totally flexible. Change positions, grab a drink, or indulge in a warm bath, and they'll likely show themselves out. It's like your body's very own rehearsal schedule.

Things worth focusing on this week

Hospital Bag Ready

It's like packing for a mini adventure, because your hospital bag is calling your name. Think of it as your ultimate survival kit for the big day. From comfy clothes to your favorite pillow, snacks, and all the essentials for both you and your baby, this bag's your backstage pass to the grand premiere of motherhood.

Rest and Recharge

Picture this – you, reclining like a queen, with your legs up for the royal treatment. Resting like a pro is now your mission. Those legs deserve some TLC, and taking moments to relax, with your feet elevated, is like giving your body the spa day it deserves.

Week 37 – 9th month–last moments :)
Your baby

Hold onto your hats, because your little champ is going full-on fat factory mode!
Your baby is in the business of gaining about 14 grams of body fat every single day. It's like they've set up shop in there, ensuring they've got the ultimate cozy insulation and a built-in snack supply.

But here's the genius part: all that baby blubber isn't just for show. It's their secret weapon for body temperature control and blood sugar mastery. It's like they're prepping for the baby Olympics of self-regulation!

And speaking of growth, let's give a round of applause to the brain and skull crew. They're not sitting around sipping baby milkshakes – they're on the move, growing and developing like the superstars they are. It's like your baby's brain is having its own personal growth spurt, getting ready to take on the world.

Your body

Baby's Descent: The Dramatic Exit Strategy
Your baby might be going for the "lowering" move on the pregnancy dance floor. Think of it as a strategic retreat, a little relief mission. With a few weeks left before the grand debut, they're taking the pressure off your lungs and diaphragm, giving you some well-deserved breathing room. It's like they're giving you a little preview of what life will be like when they finally take their bow.

Hey there, rumor mill debunker!
Let's set the record straight about the 37-week mark in this baby journey. Yes, you might have heard that at this point, the baby is labeled "undelivered," like a precious package waiting for its perfect moment.

But here's the scoop: while your little one is indeed a budding superstar, they're not quite ready to take their bow just yet. Sure, they've got that "ready for the world" look, but they're also keen on having a little extra prep time before they step onto the grand stage of life.

A chef putting the finishing touches on their gourmet meal

Those next three weeks? They're like the secret ingredients that make everything truly exquisite. Your baby's in the process of beefing up, getting those extra ounces of cuteness to keep them cozy and well-nourished.

The ultimate dynamic duo

Let's talk about the brain and lungs. They're still giving their final rehearsals before they're truly ready to shine. It's like they're practicing their moves, ensuring that when the curtain rises on the world stage, they're both well-prepared for their roles.

So, there you have it – the 37-week mark is like that exciting moment when the cake comes out of the oven, and you know it's almost time to enjoy the masterpiece. Your baby is on the brink of making their entrance, just a few more weeks of magic and preparation, and they'll be fully ready to embrace the world. It's a countdown to cuteness, and you're right at the heart of it all!

How you might feel this week?

A Breath of Fresh Air: Baby's Lowering Act

Life's all about give and take, right? Well, guess what? The good news is knocking on your pregnancy door! As your little rockstar decides to take a lower position, it's like a breath of fresh air has just entered the room – quite literally.

Say goodbye to the "baby pressing on your lungs" show, because now you can breathe easy again. It's like your lungs are throwing a party and inviting in all the oxygen they've been missing. You're back to taking those deep, satisfying breaths without feeling like you're climbing Mount Everest!

VIP Baby Zone: Lower Abdomen and Pelvis Take Center Stage

Here is the trade-off: Your lower abdomen and pelvis are the new VIP zones for your baby's presence. It's like they're making themselves comfortable, and you might just feel like there's a tiny explorer setting up camp down there. Pressure's on, but hey, it's all part of the magical journey.

The Dance of Shifting Gravity: Adjusting to New Moves

Let's talk about your center of gravity – it's taking a little detour! Your baby's descent is like a shifting spotlight, and your body's adjusting to the change. You might feel like a graceful dancer whose dance moves have been rechoreographed. Walking might feel like a gentle waltz, and balance might be giving you the tango vibes.

Things to consider

Ready, set, prepare like a pro – because you're in the final countdown to meeting your baby!
Here's your ultimate checklist for these exciting moments:

Freezer Feasts: Become a meal-prep superhero and fill that freezer with yummy, ready-to-reheat meals. Once your baby arrives, you'll be too busy enjoying the snuggles to worry about cooking. It's like stocking up on delicious life-savers for those post-baby days.

Pack like a Pro: Remember, babies are masters of surprise and only a tiny five percent stick to the scheduled due date. So, be the ultimate packing pro and have that hospital bag ready by the door. Think comfy pajamas, a snuggly bathrobe, non-slip slippers or socks for your fancy footwork, a trusty nursing bra, and all the essentials for you and your soon-to-be star.

Check and Double-Check: Your doctor's turning into a pregnancy detective, giving your cervix some serious attention. These check-ups are like the previews before the big premiere. They're keeping an eye on dilation and shortening, all those signs that your little one might be making their debut soon.
And there you have it, your pregnancy play-by-play as you gear up for the grand finale. From freezer feasts to packing prowess and doctor detective work, you've got this journey covered.

Almost There, Baby!

Guess what? Your baby's like a little overachiever, already gearing up to make their grand entrance into the world. While the official "due date" might still be a couple of weeks away, your baby's getting ready to say hello sooner than you might think. Around 85% of babies make their debut within two weeks of that date, so the countdown is on for the big moment.

Farewell to Lanugo

Imagine your baby shedding a tiny layer, like a butterfly emerging from its cocoon. That's what's happening – your baby's saying goodbye to their lanugo, that delicate layer that covered their skin for months. Some might stick around on their shoulders, forehead, or neck at birth. It's like the final touch of preparation before stepping into the world.

The Meconium Mystery

Here's a baby-sized science lesson – that lanugo and vernix? Some of it's going on an adventure, ending up in your baby's intestines. There, it becomes a key player in the formation of meconium – a greenish-black, tar-like substance. It's like the first script of your baby's life, containing traces of amniotic fluid, cells, and even snippets from their liver, pancreas, and gallbladder. This meconium will make its exit as your baby's first stool after birth.

Steady Progress

Your baby's like a little pioneer, reaching new milestones even as they prepare to make their debut. Sure, the pace might be slowing down a bit, but your baby's still on their journey of development. Each moment is like a small triumph, bringing them closer to that amazing first meeting with you.

So, mama-to-be, you're in the final chapters of this incredible story – the countdown's on, the baby's prepping, and you're getting ready to welcome them with open arms.

Enjoy every bit of this anticipation – it's like the climax before the sweetest conclusion!

Baby's Grand Entrance

Hey there, soon-to-be parent! Your baby's like a little explorer, making their way down into your pelvis – it's like their way of saying, "I'm almost ready for my debut!" While this might bring some changes, it's all part of the incredible journey.

Breathing Easier

Picture this – as your baby descends, you might notice something magical happening. You're breathing more freely, like a refreshing breeze. It's like a little gift, making this phase of your pregnancy a bit more comfortable.

Toilet Trips Galore

Now, for the not-so-surprising news – as your baby takes their position lower in your pelvis, they're also having a chit-chat with your bladder. Translation? More frequent trips to the restroom. It's like a little reminder that your baby's getting cozy for the grand entrance.

So there you have it, Mama-to-be!

How you might feel in week 38!

Fluids for Harmony

Nourishing Both of You: Picture this – your growing baby's like a little artist, creating a masterpiece of growth and development inside you. But guess what? As they grow, they're putting a bit of pressure on your bladder. It's like a friendly tap, reminding you to stay hydrated.

Imagine sipping on a refreshing drink – it's like giving your body a dose of vitality. Even though your bladder's getting a bit of a squeeze, your body still needs those fluids to stay nourished and energized.

Delivery Positions: Finding Your Comfort Zone

Remember those birthing classes where you learned all about different delivery positions? Well, now's the time to put those lessons into practice. Whether it's standing, all fours, or even rocking in a chair, it's like a mini dress rehearsal for the big day. Try out various positions at home – it's like finding your very own delivery comfort zone.

On the Road to Safety

Imagine this – you're about to embark on a journey to bring your baby home, and it's a journey you'll cherish forever. To ensure a safe and legal trip, make sure you've got a rear-facing car seat ready to go. Keep in mind that babies don't always follow schedules – they've got their own sense of timing. So, get that car seat installed early, like preparing for an adventure of a lifetime.

Baby Booties and Secret Mission Dossier

It's time to put on your superhero cape (or maybe just a comfy pair of socks) and get ready to pack your hospital bag if you haven't already! Along with the usual suspects like clothes and toiletries, don't forget to bring along some crucial documents. You'll want to have your ID, pregnancy card, info about your blood type, recent test results (especially that GBS culture), the latest ultrasound with all the juicy details about your baby's weight, and the most recent morphology report.
It's like assembling your secret mission dossier, but with more baby booties involved.

Supermom Self-Care: Recharging for Labor and Delivery

Take this time to pamper yourself and recharge those supermom batteries! Rest and relaxation are like your secret weapons to tackle the challenges of childbirth with all your might. So go ahead, put your feet up, enjoy some self-care, and get ready to rock that labor and delivery!

Week 39 – 9th month–last moments :)

Your baby

Hold onto your breath – your baby's lungs are like the ultimate construction project, gearing up for their big debut! It's like they're the superstar architects, making sure everything's in place for that magical first breath.

Surfactant Magic

Meet the secret ingredient to a perfect first breath – surfactant. Think of it as the anti-stick solution for your baby's lungs. Those air bubbles? They won't be sticking to each other, thanks to this amazing substance. It's like your baby's personal air bubble repellent, ensuring their first inhale is as smooth as can be.

Stress Hormone Showdown

Get ready for a hormone showdown – your baby's secretory system is like the star of this drama. During labor, it releases more stress hormones than at any other time in their life. But here's the twist – these hormones are like the ultimate helpers. Once your baby's out in the world, they'll kick in, managing their body systems without the placenta's backup. It's like their grand finale, full of energy and effort.

Lung Symphony

Imagine your baby's lungs as an orchestra, tuning up for the performance of a lifetime. From development to surfactant production, it's like they're composing the perfect melody for that first breath-taking note.

Your body

Mama's Blood: The Ultimate Baby Bodyguard

Get ready for a mind-blowing fact, Mama – your blood is like the ultimate gift of protection for your baby! As it circulates through the placenta, it's like passing on a treasure trove of antibodies, all set to help your little one fight infections after they make their grand entrance into the world. Imagine this: your blood's like a superhero squad, equipped with all the tools to keep your baby safe.

Those antibodies?

They're like the ultimate defenders, ready to jump into action when needed. It's like giving your baby a head start in the immunity game, making sure they're well-prepared for the adventures that await them. So, as your body continues its incredible journey, remember that you're not just nurturing your baby – you're also passing on a shield of protection, a gift that'll stay with them and support them as they step into the world.

How you might feel in week 39?

Contractions: The Dress Rehearsal and the Grand Entrance

You've got your pregnancy detective hat on, and you're sorting out those contractions like a pro. If you notice contractions that are irregular and seem to ease up when you switch positions or take a walk, you're likely experiencing Braxton Hicks contractions. They're like your body's dress rehearsal for the big show.

But here's the twist – things can change in the blink of an eye. Those "practice" contractions might suddenly decide it's showtime and transform into the real deal. It's like your body's way of surprising you with a grand entrance!

Keep your eyes on the clock – it's your secret weapon.

When those contractions start playing tag and show up at regular intervals, like every five minutes, and keep it up for at least an hour, that's your cue to pick up the phone. Call your doctor, midwife, or nurse – they're like your backstage crew, ready to guide you through this amazing journey.

And hey, if the waters decide to make a dramatic exit, consider that your spotlight moment has officially arrived.

Things to consider

Contraction Chronicles: It's like you're the official contractions timekeeper. Measure each one with precision, making sure not to raise the false alarm flag. It's all about being the captain of the contraction ship, ready to navigate through the real deal and the practice rounds.

Name Game: Drumroll, please – the baby's name is like the ultimate starring role in this show. Make that final decision, because soon enough, your baby's going to rock that name like a true superstar. It's like giving them their very own identity, a name that'll be music to your ears for a lifetime.

Mom-to-Mom Chats: Imagine this – you and fellow moms, gathered around like a circle of wisdom. Talking about positive birth experiences is like a treasure hunt for tips, insights, and a dose of confidence. It's like tapping into a sisterhood of support, getting you all geared up for your own amazing story.

Bag of Wonders: Your hospital bag is like the ultimate adventure kit, ready to roll at a moment's notice. It's packed with everything you need, like a treasure chest of essentials for both you and your baby. Imagine grabbing that bag and knowing you're fully prepared for the magical moment ahead.

Week 40 – OMG! It is happening!
Your baby

Baby's Extended Stay: The Luxury Vacation Inside

As you eagerly anticipate the arrival of your newest family member, your little one might decide to extend their luxury vacation within your belly for a few more days or even weeks (oh, the nerve!).

If that's the case, your doctor will be on standby, closely checking your baby's weight gain and their opinion on contractions – you know, the usual chit-chat.

Spinning Babies and Cesarean Chats

Your baby's got a cozy spot, all curled up, in your womb. But hold onto your hats – if they're feeling a bit adventurous and choose a breech position (feet or bottom first), the doctor might just play tour guide and try to spin them around. If that doesn't quite work out like a fancy dance move, brace yourself for a sit-down discussion about a potential cesarean section – because life's all about keeping things interesting!

Baby's Birth Stats: Chunky, Cozy, and Ready to Roll!

Well, congrats, because your little VIP is likely done fine-tuning his birth stats – weight and height, all locked and loaded! About 15% of that adorable chunkiness is pure baby blubber, designed to keep him cozy and snug in the big wide world. Think of it as his built-in snuggle buddy.

We're Open for business

Organs, check. Body systems, check. Even his liver has been playing starchy banker, stocking up on glucose for the post-womb adventure. And if that's not enough, he's got some hydration tricks up his sleeve too, like a little baby camel.

Ready for the ultimate symphony?

Hold your breath for that very first cry! But hey, did you know your mini-me won't be shedding any heart-wrenching tears for about a month? Those tiny tear ducts need a bit of time to unclog and unleash the waterworks.

A Magical Measuring Tape and Early Arrival Prowess!

And here's a fun surprise – your baby's actual age might throw you a curveball. After the grand debut, a nurse or pediatrician will whip out their magical measuring tape and neurological crystal ball to estimate his "true" age based on appearance and development. It's like their way of giving a thumbs-up to his readiness for the outside world. So, prepare for some "age-difference" shenanigans as your baby dazzles you with his early arrival prowess!

Your body

The Countdown Continues

Hey there, soon-to-be parent! Your baby's like a little secret agent, orchestrating their grand entrance on their own schedule. While you're eagerly awaiting the face-to-face introduction, let's talk about these last few days – they're like a treasure trove of opportunities to spoil yourself a bit.

Savor the Me-Time

Imagine this – it's like you're about to embark on a thrilling adventure, and these days are like a cozy prelude. Indulge yourself with the little things that bring joy – maybe a relaxing pedicure, a captivating movie marathon, or getting lost in a book cover to cover. It's like creating a sanctuary of "you" time before the whirlwind of baby care begins.

A Date with Yourself

Picture this – once your bundle of joy arrives, you'll be on your toes, 24/7. So, consider these moments a special date with yourself. It's like collecting these memories as gems to treasure during the busy days ahead.

How you might feel this week?

The Grand Finale

Congratulations, mama-to-be!

You're on the threshold of an incredible journey – the labor of love that will bring your precious baby into the world. But how do you know when the show's about to begin? Let's talk about the telltale signs.

Contractions Take Center Stage

Imagine this – it's like your body's putting on a performance, and contractions are the stars of the show. Look out for regular contractions that start mild, then gradually become stronger and longer over time. It's like the prelude to the most incredible act.

Mucus Magic

Picture this – your body's got a few tricks up its sleeve, and one of them is the "mucus plug" or "labor plug." It's like nature's way of saying, "Get ready, we're getting close!" Keep an eye out for this discharge from your vagina.

Waters in Motion

Now, here comes the dramatic moment – the "rupture of the membranes." Imagine it as a water show, where the amniotic fluid breaks free. It's like the opening act of the grand finale.

Doctor's Advice

Hey, when in doubt, reach out to your doctor. They're like the directors guiding you through this incredible performance. If you spot any of those "uh-oh" signs, it's their cue to step in and guide you.

Home Sweet Home

Now, here's a little twist in the plot, Mama – as the spotlight's about to shine on you, you might feel the urge to rush to the hospital. But hold your applause for a moment. Consider this – basking in the excitement at home might just be the perfect build-up to the grand finale.

Things to consider this last week

Bag at the Ready, Captain!

Imagine this – your hospital bag is practically tapping its fingers, waiting oh-so-patiently for its moment in the spotlight. It's like the most eager contestant in the "Ready-to-Go Olympics."

Oh, Just Any Day Now!

Well, isn't that just the most precise timeframe ever? Your little nugget is like a super punctual party guest – showing up whenever they feel like it.

Best Of Luck Mama, You Got This!

Table of Contents